FOREVER Painless

Also by MIRANDA ESMONDE-WHITE

Aging Backwards

FOREVER
Painless

END CHRONIC PAIN AND
RECLAIM YOUR LIFE IN
30 MINUTES A DAY

Miranda Esmonde-White

HARPER WAVE

An Imprint of HarperCollins*Publishers*

This book contains advice and information relating to health care. It should be used to supplement rather than replace the advice of your doctor or another trained health professional. If you know or suspect you have a health problem, it is recommended that you seek your physician's advice before embarking on any medical program or treatment. All efforts have been made to ensure the accuracy of the information contained in this book as of the date of publication. This publisher and the author disclaim liability for any medical outcomes that may occur as a result of applying the methods suggested in this book.

HarperCollins books may be purchased for educational, business, or sales promotional use. For information, please email the Special Markets Department at SPsales@harpercollins.com.

FIRST EDITION

Designed by Leah Carlson-Stanisic

Exercise photos in chapters 6 and 9 by Alexandre Paskanoi. All other exercise photos by Allison Flam.

Library of Congress Cataloging-in-Publication Data has been applied for.

ISBN 978-0-06-244866-8

16 17 18 19 20 RRD 10 9 8 7 6 5 4 3 2 1

This book is dedicated to my daughter, Sahra Esmonde-White, and all the hardworking staff at the Essentrics office who made it possible.

Contents

Foreword

Chronic pain can result from many different causes, but once pain becomes chronic, life becomes very difficult. One of the most damaging consequences of pain, whatever or wherever its origin, is the tendency to stop moving. We stop moving because it hurts to move, or because we fear that movement will make things worse, or because we're too exhausted even to think about moving. But the reality is that being sedentary only worsens chronic pain, and initiates a downward spiral that prevents us from recovering: As we move less, our muscles become weak, our connective tissues stiffen, our posture deteriorates, and our stamina decreases. Consequently, any type of physical activity becomes even more difficult. On the other end of the spectrum, programs that encourage people to "push through the pain" with repetitive exercises cause muscle strain and inflammation, prolonging chronic pain and making it worse. Soon discouragement sets in.

With her deceptively simple exercise program, Essentrics, Miranda Esmonde-White offers a hopeful alternative for the millions of people who suffer from chronic pain. Essentrics uses a simple technique that can gently interrupt and reverse the cycle of pain and physical deterioration. The beauty of the program is its balance of stretching, strengthening, posture, and cardiovascular work. Most important, it leaves no stone unturned, as every part of the body from the fingers to the toes receives attention, restoring harmony and bringing the body back in tune with itself. The emphasis on relaxing tight muscles while performing whole-body movements allows more and more of the body to participate, as tight and painful areas are able to let go and stop sending pain signals.

In my personal experience of doing Miranda's program for the past three years, I have become noticeably stronger and more flexible, never once experiencing any aggravation of pain the day after a workout. This is significant for me, as I have a long history of chronic pain. For more than twenty years, every physical treatment or exercise I ever tried either did not work or made the pain worse. But after doing this program, my chronic pain is now gone.

To develop Essentrics, Miranda Esmonde-White used her basic training in classical ballet as a starting point, and supplemented it with conventional physiotherapy, tai chi, and a wide variety of other disciplines she had gleaned from her lifelong studies. In her popular public television series *Classical Stretch*, which has been on the air since 1999, she is a delightful coach, encouraging and coaxing viewers with grace and humor. Just watching her move so beautifully, even when she is well into her sixties, is an inspiration. Now in this book, she explains in detail the rationale underlying her exercise program and how it may benefit anyone who suffers from chronic musculoskeletal pain.

My own research on connective tissue suggests that gentle stretching is an essential part of any treatment protocol for chronic pain, as it reduces inflammation and helps heal injuries. Essentrics exercises are gentle but powerful, and come with the explicit instruction to go slowly and change "one cell at a time." This is an especially important point when it comes to working with our connective tissues, also known as fascia, which can easily be injured by excessive or rapid stretching.

I look forward to the day when we will have a research study that measures the effects of Miranda's incredible program. In the meantime, we are fortunate to have this treasure of a book, and it is up to each of us to make use of it.

> Helene M. Langevin, MD
> Professor in Residence of Medicine
> Director, Osher Center for Integrative Medicine
> Brigham and Women's Hospital, Harvard Medical School

Introduction

The experience of pain can disrupt our lives on a day-to-day, minute-to-minute basis. The amount of mental, emotional, and physical energy necessary to battle chronic pain can leave us exhausted and demoralized, with little hope for relief. Relationships suffer; jobs are lost. Pain limits our possibilities, shrinks our world, clouds our perceptions, and leaves us less engaged with our families and in our lives.

But when we're able to find relief from pain, the whole world changes. Once fearful of movement, we can return to and enjoy our favorite activities, from taking long walks to playing tennis to running around with our children or grandchildren. Without the mental and physical distraction of pain plaguing us, we can be present and enjoy our time with loved ones. We can forgo dependence on others and reclaim our independence, our freedom. We can once again carry our own groceries, walk up and down stairs, and tend to our own gardens. Our lives, once dimmed by pain, become brighter and full of promise.

Sound too good to be true? It's not. I promise you, healing from chronic pain—an actual cure for your pain—*is* possible. Unfortunately, the current medical approach to treating pain is not to heal it, but to *manage* it. Chronic pain is seen as something to be minimized or muted or coped with, rather than to be permanently fixed. In an effort to rescue their patients from pain, many doctors' primary focus has been on providing immediate relief through pharmaceuticals. But we now know that short-term solutions, though temporarily effective, carry tremendous risk.

Today America is in the midst of an opioid addiction epidemic that has quadrupled in the last decade, claiming lives on a minute-by-minute basis. Drug overdoses have become the leading cause of accidental death in the United States, and opioids have driven this epidemic. In 2014 alone, almost nineteen thousand overdose deaths were linked to prescription pain relievers—almost twice as many deaths as those linked to heroin.[1] Despite their widespread use, opioids provide only fleeting relief from pain, with patients quickly building up a tolerance. Our quest for a quick fix has left us in the midst of an ever more dangerous public health crisis and, tragically, much further from the true pain cure we need.

Thankfully, in recent years, neurologists have begun to uncover evidence that we can, indeed, heal from pain—not just block it or mask it. And as with many forms of healing, the most powerful natural remedy does not come in the form of a pill—it comes from within our own bodies.

Correct Exercise Is the Silver Bullet

We know that we need to exercise to stay fit. Your doctors have likely encouraged you to exercise regularly—but their suggestions were probably focused on promoting heart health, balancing your blood sugar, or helping you lose a few pounds. We are told, simply, that exercise is good—we should all just do *some* exercise, *any* exercise, to remain healthy. However, such general recommendations do nothing to *address* the issue of healing pain. In fact, though this guidance may be well intentioned, the lack of specificity is a problem. When exercise programs are taken to an extreme, they are often counterproductive, aging the body and laying the foundation for chronic pain.

It's time for a new approach. We need to recognize that *how* we exercise matters. Rather than unquestioningly follow the *anything-is-better-than-nothing* approach, we need to be very conscious of what type of exercise we're prescribing for ourselves. We need a complete mind shift around movement.

To heal our pain, stay youthful and limber, and prevent premature aging, we need to focus on exercises that refresh our tissues and reawaken our cells. Such movements can help us maintain peak function throughout our lives—not just in our youth. We need to put a high premium on balance, clean alignment, muscle strength, and full connective tissue mobility. To make it accessible to everyone, this approach should also be very simple: it should require little to no equipment; use only a small amount of space; and be versatile enough to be done anytime, anywhere. If we can incorporate this type of exercise program into our daily lives, we should be able not only to help our heart, reduce our blood sugar, and maybe shed a few pounds but also to *reverse* age-related decline, *heal* our bodies, and *cure* our chronic pain.

Essentrics—the method of dynamic stretching and strengthening that I have taught to millions of people with my PBS show, *Classical Stretch*, can do just that. I first created the Essentrics technique to heal my own chronic pain. As it has evolved, Essentrics has been influenced by several disciplines, drawing on the flowing movements of tai chi to create health and balance; the strengthening theories of ballet to create long, lean, flexible muscles; and the healing principles of physical therapy and scientific studies to create a pain-free body.

One of the greatest joys of my life is teaching people the Essentrics method and watching them reemerge into the light from the cloud of chronic pain. The Essentrics method uses "eccentric" exercises—those that simultaneously strengthen and lengthen muscle—to rebalance the body's muscular structure through continuous rotational movements. It incorporates various techniques while systematically working every joint in the body. The basis of the workout is a dynamic combination of strength and flexibility exercises designed to gently open the joints by elongating the muscles and challenging them in the lengthened position. This full-body technique works through the muscle chains, liberating and empowering the muscles, relieving them from tension in the process.

Essentrics workouts—comprised of deliberate, focused movements done in a specific sequence—can unlock long-standing knots, rebuild flexibility into stiffened joints, and reduce all types of musculoskeletal and myofascial pain. While I've known for years that Essentrics can sometimes trigger spontaneous healing of pain, we were never quite certain of the mechanisms involved. But recent studies have revealed that Essentrics is able to heal pain by tapping into a previously unknown pathway that flows directly through the fascia—the connective tissue—itself.

Researchers now know that fascia, once thought to function simply as the packing material that holds the body together, plays a much more significant role in the body, transmitting messages of pain or pleasure, tension or relaxation, inflammation or healing. Chinese medicine recognized this principle two thousand years ago with the introduction of acupuncture, still one of the most effective natural remedies for pain relief. Today, it's been proved that Essentrics taps into this innate whole-body healing network, sending healing messages to various body systems at once. In fact, thanks to its full-body rebalancing approach, Essentrics may trigger the very same self-healing mechanisms in the body that acupuncture does—but without the needles!

Regardless of whether or not we will eventually be able to pinpoint the exact mechanisms involved in the healing process, the most important thing to know about Essentrics is something I have known—and witnessed firsthand—for decades: It often *cures* pain. And when used consistently, Essentrics allows us to rebuild lost strength, to regain hope, and to remain sustainably pain-free for the rest of our lives without dependence on drugs or expensive medical treatments.

I do want to be clear: if the joint degeneration is extreme, as in the case of advanced arthritis, *complete* pain relief may not be possible. However, some degree of pain relief likely can be achieved by decompressing the joint through stretching and strengthening. We can rebuild muscle strength and flexibility—but sadly, we cannot rebuild destroyed bone.

Our bodies hold the most powerful, versatile, and effective keys to unlocking our pain—we just need to know how to use them.

What This Book Will Do for You

This book will help you understand what might be causing your pain so that you can begin to cure it. It will also teach you how your cells, connective tissue, blood, muscles, and joints react when you do the right exercise, the wrong exercise, or—the worst—no exercise.

In part 1, you'll learn how people have been misunderstanding and thus perpetuating pain for decades. I'll talk about some of the most common causes of pain, many of which we bring upon ourselves. You'll learn about the groundbreaking research that's revolutionizing our understanding of chronic pain. And you'll see why a well-constructed rebalancing exercise program—not a dangerous drug or medical treatment—is the *only* sustainable, healthy, and effective means to *permanently* prevent and alleviate many types of pain.

Part 2 offers detailed exercise workouts designed to heal the body of specific types of chronic pains. Chapter 5 presents a basic warm-up routine that must not be overlooked—it is essential to warm up properly before you begin any workout. Next you'll make your way through several sequences of movements, each targeted to heal a particular area of the body. While these routines are meant to address specific pain pathways, you'll find that they are often appropriate for other types of pain within each region. For example, while ten different people may have ten different causes of hip pain, similar exercises can be helpful for each. A hip is a hip—it has a torso on top and legs underneath! The hips all work with the same muscles, tendons, ligaments, joints, and connective tissue. An Essentrics hip-pain workout rebalances the full anatomical structure of the hip, so it addresses the various causes of pain simultaneously. Chapters 6 to 14 offer specific routines for pain associated with certain body parts such as knees, hips, backs, and shoulders, or for conditions that cause pain, like fibromyalgia or arthritis. All the exercises in part 2 are drawn from the Essentrics technique, and all have been successfully used by tens of thousands of people to relieve their pain.

Along the way, you'll also read stories from people like you who suffered from chronic pain and have found lasting relief using Essentrics. You may find yourself relating to or empathizing with their years of suffering. My hope is that you'll also find inspiration and encouragement in their perseverance. Their dramatic experiences show us that real relief from chronic pain is within reach.

For almost two decades, it has been my mission to help people live vibrant, pain-free lives at every age. When we understand what's going on inside our bodies, we are able to make clear decisions about how to keep ourselves pain-free, healthy, and vital. No matter what your age, no matter how long you've been in pain, I believe you can heal. I believe you can be free. I believe Essentrics can help you be painless, forever.

Part One

When the Pain Doesn't Go Away

CHAPTER 1

Our Modern Epidemic of Pain

Pain is part of the human condition. During our lifetimes, we all experience a few episodes of acute physical pain. Not many of us will escape the kind of pain we feel after stubbing a toe, spraining an ankle, or stepping barefoot on a piece of glass. But fortunately, for most people, acute pain tends to be as short-lived as it is severe.

This type of pain is normal; it's healthy pain. Healthy pain is an indicator that something is wrong or is doing damage to our body. Healthy pain is part of an essential warning system—without feeling the sharp pain that accompanies a broken limb, for example, we would carry on using it until we caused even greater damage. So in situations of injury, pain functions as a protective alarm, warning us that our house is on fire and we must take action to save it. Once the fire is out—once the broken bone has healed or the torn muscle repaired—the pain should recede.

This acute pain is completely different from the type of pain that comprises four of the top 10 reasons why Americans consult doctors and other health-care providers: chronic pain. Often, chronic pain is the fire alarm that won't shut off. This enduring, unrelieved pain is a major global health-care problem, a disease in its own right. For sometimes mysterious reasons, this pain may start gently but, over time, become stronger and stronger. We might visit several different doctors in our search for the cause of the pain, but the

PAIN AND DEPRESSION: A TWO-WAY STREET

Pain and depression tend to go together, for both biological and psychological reasons. When you're in pain, you understandably tend to feel more depressed; when you are depressed, your body actually has a heightened sensitivity to pain. The factors involved are complex and often misunderstood. For example, imbalances in certain neurotransmitters, such as serotonin and norepinephrine, are linked to both depression and pain—a fact that can lead some to believe "it's all in the head."[1] But both conditions are also characterized by systemic inflammation, a risk factor for heart disease, diabetes, and many autoimmune conditions. And research has proved that the worse our painful physical symptoms are, the more severe any related depression tends to be.[2]

We need to take this connection extremely seriously. In a recent review in the journal *Current Psychiatry Reports*, Scottish researchers found that up to 50 percent of chronic pain patients also suffered from depression related to the pain, and 17 percent suffered so badly that some days they wanted to die.[3] A Canadian study found that people living with pain had double the risk of suicide, compared with people without chronic pain.[4]

These statistics are tragic to me. People need help, right now.

The program in this book can help you recover both mentally and physically; exercise is a proven remedy for both pain and depression. But please be gentle with yourself and realize that sometimes exercise is not enough. Be sure to talk about your physical and emotional health with your doctor; getting the help you need for either pain or depression will automatically help both.

truth is, many times the root cause is easily overlooked. It may be something as simple as sitting hunched in front of a computer all day. Or that bicycle accident we had a decade ago. Or something else—we often just don't know.

None of the standard medical approaches are designed to permanently relieve non-disease-related chronic pain. It seems to persist even with visits to massage therapists, physical therapists, osteopaths, chiropractors, and other specialists. These passive treatments feel good and provide temporary relief—but the pain usually returns within hours.

According to the National Institutes of Health, chronic pain is the most common cause of long-term disability in the United States. Chronic pain is a life-altering, life-limiting daily state for one in five U.S. adults. The American Chronic Pain Association lists lower back problems, arthritis, repetitive stress injuries, headaches, and fibromyalgia as some of the most common sources of pain.

The price tag of chronic pain is staggering. In the United States, the cost of chronic pain in adults, including health-care expenses and lost productivity, has been estimated at $560 billion to $630 billion annually. (That's *billion* with a *b*!) Then there is the incalculable toll on individuals and families. A survey of almost fifty thousand Europeans found that 27 percent of chronic pain sufferers said their pain made maintaining their relationships with family and friends very difficult, if not impossible.[5] Chronic pain sufferers experience deficits in all kinds of cognitive functioning, including perception, thinking, reasoning, and memory. According to the *European Journal of Pain*, 61 percent of those with chronic pain are less able or simply unable to work outside the home because of their pain.[6] One Canadian study found that arthritis pain shortened sufferers' working lives by an average of four years.[7]

Sadly, due to their inability to diagnose or treat so-called mechanical pain (or nonspecific musculoskeletal pain), many doctors believe that some degree of pain is normal and that we should be prepared to tolerate it. And millions of people do just that, year after year. Too often people turn to doctors who have little training in pain management and who tend to freely prescribe drugs, including opioids, in response to complaints of pain. Even if you put aside the serious risk of overdose and death, opioids can also increase the risk of accidents, disrupt your periods (if you're a woman), lower your sex drive (whether you're a woman or a man), trigger sleep apnea, cause constipation, and contribute to heart and lung problems. Many doctors simply aren't educated about the risks. In fact, a recent Canadian study found that veterinarians receive *five times more training* in pain management than medical doctors do.[8] And a European survey of patients suffering moderate to severe chronic pain found that one in four patients said their doctor never asked about pain or, if pain was discussed, the doctor did not know how to treat it.

I am not a doctor—but I am a firm believer that the topic of pain should be a routine part of our health checkups, and that we should expect our doctors to be able to offer solutions beyond medication. Living pain-free should be a human right. The preamble to the World Health Organization's constitution—which was adopted in 1948 and has remained unchanged ever since—defines *health* as "a state of complete physical, mental and social well-being and not merely the absence of disease or infirmity."[9] I agree wholeheartedly with this view—it's the only way that pain is going to get the respect, attention, medical research, and treatment options it deserves. Unfortunately, many research dollars dedicated to investigating pain are focused on pharmaceuticals, not long-term relief. But we don't have to wait for the medical establishment to catch up—we already have plenty of evidence that our bodies hold the keys to a pain-free life.

Our Body's Built-In Pain Relief

Traditional approaches to anatomy and health have taught us that the human body is the sum total of many independent systems:

The brain and nerves function as our nervous system.

Muscles, bones, and soft tissues comprise our musculoskeletal system.

The glands and organs that regulate our hormones make up our endocrine system.

The heart and blood vessels, which pump blood and oxygen to every cell in the body, form the cardiovascular system.

The organ systems, combined, are the engines of life.

Every moment of our lives depends on the complex interaction of these systems. And for a long time, the connective-tissue system—the bands and sheets of fascia under the skin that attach, enclose, and separate our muscles and organs—were seen as the supporting structure for the other systems, which did the *real* work of keeping us alive and healthy. But the more we learn about the integral role that fascia plays in our overall health, the more we're starting to see that the best way to keep all of these systems functioning properly is to keep connective tissue healthy, strong, and flexible. The closest thing that we have to a universal cure-all is *regular exercise with correct form*.

Every bite of food we eat and every thought we think creates a ripple effect within the body. We know that if we eat refined carbohydrates, for example, our pancreas will release more insulin to help our cells absorb the sudden increase in blood sugar. On the flip side, we also know that if we take a moment to pause amid a stressful day to take a few deep breaths, our circulatory system will carry extra-oxygenated blood up to the brain and to all of our muscles, helping us feel calmer, sharper, and more energized.

In much the same way, each time we twist or turn, bend or lift, the stretching triggers changes in our connective tissue, and different messages start careening throughout our body. Doctors used to believe that many of these messages were carried exclusively by the nervous system, but new theories suggest that connective tissue also plays a critical role in this messaging network. Because not only does our connective tissue support our musculoskeletal system, it also provides the actual building blocks of our organs. Researchers now believe that this tissue could function as its own "meta-system" within the body, constantly connecting with various regions and coordinating the messages and activities of each bodily system.

Most of us have never given much thought to our fascia. We may have a vague idea that fascia fills in the gaps in our body, but new research suggests that this connective tissue is not passive at all. Recent studies by Dr. Helene M. Langevin, director of the Osher Center for Integrative Medicine (jointly based at Brigham and Women's Hospital and Harvard Medical School) and a professor of neurological sciences at the University of Vermont, have found that connective tissue not only lengthens and changes in response to pressure from the outside—such as stretching or the insertion of acupuncture needles—but also lengthens and reorganizes itself from within. Dr. Langevin's studies have shown that when needles are inserted into the collagen of the fascia during acupuncture, connective tissue "grabs" the needle and twists around it. Then, a few moments later, fascial cells located a few centimeters away from the needle extend and fundamentally change their composition in response.

Let's take a moment to let that sink in: not only is this tissue being moved by an outside force—it is also *moving and stretching and changing itself from within.*[10] Amazing, right? The idea of self-stretching tissue suddenly makes our fascia seem a lot more active and dynamic—and essential to our health—than we once assumed.

While it's incredible that connective tissue has the ability to react to movement, the only way to trigger this self-healing reaction is just that: with movement. The more we learn about Essentrics, the clearer it becomes that this type of exercise is exactly what our connective tissue needs to facilitate internal changes. And perhaps most exciting of all is the idea that these changes may actually be a self-healing mechanism that the scientific community has been trying to pinpoint for centuries.

Sound far-fetched? Consider some other self-healing mechanisms in the human body that we take for granted:

If we cut ourselves, the wound will eventually close and the skin will grow back.

If we break a bone, it will fuse itself back together once it is set properly.

If we get a cold or the flu, our immune system will send in white blood cells to fight off pathogens and we'll recover after a week or two.

We know that our body holds the ability to heal itself. And we also know there are things we can do to help support its healing processes, and things we can do to hurt it. We know that if we slather a cut with an ointment and cover it with a bandage, we'll protect it from infection. We know that if we rest and elevate a broken bone, allowing our circulatory system to carry nutrients and waste products to and from the site of the injury, it will heal faster. We know that if we eat healthy foods and drink plenty of water, we'll give our immune system the tools it needs to fight off viruses or bacteria.

We take all this for granted—but we haven't made the same connection between movement and healing our pain. We don't yet fully realize the power we have to control and cure our own pain. Just as we can encourage our body's other self-healing processes through small steps of self-care, so too can we encourage the body's pain-healing processes with small doses of gentle movement.

When you understand how the body works, even on the most basic level, you see how the choices we make can either accelerate or prevent healing. I believe so much of the chronic pain that people are suffering right now could be greatly reduced or eliminated simply by understanding how we can tap into these self-healing mechanisms with gentle, correct exercises. Not only will this help us stay vital during our normal life span, but by practicing specific exercises, we can continue to extend that life span far beyond the one we've come to see as normal. But we must act *now*—without proper exercise, our life span may actually be shrinking, due to our current lifestyle choices.

Pain Can Age Us

We see the signs of "normal" aging all around us—poor posture, lack of energy, diminished vibrancy, unexplained weight gain, osteoporosis, arthritis, and chronic pain. Most of us—including myself, until recently—have begrudgingly accepted chronic pain and muscular atrophy as normal parts of aging. But now we know better: Neither chronic pain nor premature aging (which is often caused by pain) is really normal. Both can be greatly prevented with simple movement.

In my first book, *Aging Backwards*, I described the results of a groundbreaking study conducted at the University of Pittsburgh in 2011. Using MRI measurements of the muscle tissue in forty high-level athletes, researchers discovered that the lean muscle tissue of a seventy-four-year-old triathlete was *exactly the same* as the lean muscle tissue of a forty-year-old triathlete with a similar exercise program. The study showed that one of the primary markers of aging—loss of muscle mass—could be completely controlled by movement, and thus that loss of muscle mass is *not* a guaranteed fact of aging. In fact, the researchers discovered that what was previously considered aging was actually just muscle atrophy.

This study proved my long-standing belief: We are only as old as our muscles are inactive.

A lack of full-body movement tells our cells that they are no longer needed, setting off a chain reaction of cell death. This domino effect gradually impacts all of our bodily systems, weakening our muscles and shutting down our major organ systems prematurely. But if we use the right types of exercise to maintain our muscle mass into our later years, our entire bodies—even those pesky joints that typically fail us first—can stay healthy until we are well over one hundred years old.

But when we do the wrong exercise—well, that can be almost as bad as not exercising at all.

When Exercise Ages Us

Movement is a gift, our very own personal health-care system. Yet because our culture has not traditionally recognized the absolute necessity of movement in the essential maintenance of life, we approach exercise in a disjointed and uneducated fashion. Because we have a limited scientific understanding of what our bodies receive from us when we exercise, we tend to follow a Wild West approach. Some people do a lot of exercise; others do none. Some people follow the fitness fads; others just do whatever their friends are doing. Some people even choose the most challenging program available and train like maniacs, believing that their hard work will reward them with peak physical fitness.

The gung-ho approach may seem consequence-free when we are young and relatively fearless in our twenties and thirties. This means that, unless we learn how to properly exercise early on in our youth, we are innocently yet actively injuring ourselves, aging our cells, atrophying our muscles, literally shrinking away—without even knowing it.

From a diagnostic perspective, it is often impossible to understand why one person is in pain while someone with the identical condition is not. To make matters even more confusing, consider this: There are some people whose X-rays indicate major spinal degeneration, and who normally would be in pain but are in fact pain-free; however, there are others who express extreme pain but have X-rays indicating no spinal degeneration. A possible explanation in the subjective experience of pain may be linked to the fact that some people have more or fewer nociceptors, sensory nerve cells that form the basis of the pain messaging system. Other differences in pain perception are related to levels of depression or stress (see page 4 for more information).

But over the course of a lifetime, no one is immune from pain.

Through our many years, we will inevitably get sick, break a bone, or twist an ankle. We will all experience some degree of illness and pain. And as we know, acute pain is a normal, healthy signal of distress in the body. Yet we should certainly never consider it "normal" to endure chronic pain for months or years. Nothing ages us faster than constant pain and suffering.

Before we let ourselves feel the first creak or ache, we should start protecting our bodies with correct exercise. But even after decades of pounding your joints in intense workouts, Essentrics can help turn back the clock on your body—and turn down the dial on your pain.

The Essentrics Difference

With our fragmented approach to health, we often forget that the body is one unit, and every cell—from blood to nerve, from skin to bone—is talking to every other cell, all at the same time. The simple and profound brilliance of our body's interconnectivity cannot be overstated: Everything we do, both right and wrong, is registered in our body. Every movement counts. When we truly accept and understand this, we can make simple changes that will help us maintain vibrant, healthy bodies; but when we ignore this, we are at the mercy of accelerated cell death and a possible future of chronic pain.

Knowledge gives us a choice: we can begin to completely reroute our body's destiny with just a few small changes. And that's what I want to share in this book—the knowledge that will set you free from your pain. The Essentrics program is scientifically designed to keep our bodies well balanced and healthy at any age. The exercises are easy to do, take only about 30 minutes a day, and are appropriate for anyone who is seeking a drug-free, sustainable approach to pain relief. Unlike pharmaceuticals, my program has side effects that are actually beneficial and health-promoting: lowered stress; increased energy, strength, and endurance; improved mood; better sleep; and greater physical flexibility. People at any level of fitness—from those who've become completely sedentary to elite world-class athletes—have found tremendous pain-relief benefit from Essentrics.

Are you surprised to hear that both completely inactive and highly active people can use the exact same program to get results? Well, here's the dirty secret about a long-held yet mistaken belief that continues to infect the fitness field: The classic "no pain, no gain" approach should be abandoned in favor of "any pain, no gain." Imbalanced physical activity has left many avid athletes nearly incapacitated in middle age. Imbalanced muscles are a universal risk factor for pain, whether you're a new mother who carries her ten-pound diaper bag on only one shoulder or a competitive bodybuilder whose massive pectorals are the envy of the gym.

The Essentrics approach is "no pain, ever." By following a program whose main focus is correcting imbalanced muscles, you can teach your body how to do all the activities you love to do more easily and fluidly, without ever holding on to pain. Active people can continue to enjoy sports like skiing, golf, or tennis for as long as they like, pain-free. Formerly sedentary people can regain the joy of movement, heal their back or sciatic pain, and build endurance. Overworked executives can release tension headaches and shoulder pain, and have more stamina and mental acuity. With these exercises, anyone can

A FEW CAVEATS

While we will all experience pain at some point in our lives, everyone's pain is unique. There are some types of pain that Essentrics is not able to address—namely, pain caused by congenital, genetic, or other non-lifestyle-based diseases.

While I am evangelical about the healing power of correct movement, I also know that there are many afflictions for which movement is not enough. Many diseases are painful—of course they are! Pain is the body's message, warning us that something is wrong. There are many diseases that arise from chemical "imbalance"—such as cancer, inflammatory conditions, blood disorders, and organ failures—that cause extreme pain. Exercising cannot cure this type of pain, as it is not caused by mechanical flaws.

In fact, most disease is not mechanical, but chemical. And as far as we know now, exercise works on the mechanics of the body, not the chemistry. But research is digging into potential mechanisms that might bridge this mechanical-chemical gap, and we may soon learn exactly how exercise can, in fact, help prevent and even cure some chemically based diseases. So stay tuned to these studies becoming more public. But for now, please understand that pain related to chemically based disease must be relieved through treatments given by medical specialists, not fitness instructors. (See the appendix for other healing modalities that can help relieve pain.)

continue to safely participate in the activity of his or her choice—simply by maintaining a well-balanced body in 30 minutes a day.

These were lessons I had to learn for myself—the hard way. I, too, have a long personal history of chronic pain. It was only after I'd turned forty that I began to experience the painful toll of the many years I'd spent as a professional ballet dancer. In response to my own pain, I created this approach—and since then, I have been pain-free. As I write this book, I am sixty-six, and I feel even fitter than I did in my thirties. I never want to go back to those years of chronic pain—and, thanks to the gift of Essentrics, I know I never have to.

Exercise Is Medicine

When I developed Essentrics, my objective was to create a safer, gentler, less aggressive method of becoming fit by providing an alternative to the hard-core workouts that had permeated the market—and still do! As a technique, Essentrics is the antithesis of pumping iron and pounding the pavement; it's slow and gentle, simultaneously stretching and strengthening all 650 muscles in the body as it rebalances all 384 joints.

Almost immediately after I began teaching this method, my first group of students began to share what have since become its two most often cited benefits: *I feel so much younger when I do this* and *I don't feel as much pain when I do this*. Fast-forward almost two decades, and the combination of anti-aging and pain relief has become the sole focus of my life. Over that time, I've seen firsthand how Essentrics relieves the most common pain conditions that are presumed to be related to aging: back pain, plantar fasciitis, fibromyalgia, arthritis, and osteoporosis, among many others.

Now, after teaching and hearing from thousands of pain-free students, I have become that much more convinced that the chronic pain that plagues millions worldwide is completely unnecessary. All we need to do is give the body what it needs: a short, gentle, daily workout of pleasurable lengthening and strengthening movements. That's it!

The human body is a very complex machine, but in its purest state, it is designed to be free of pain. Let's take a closer look at our fascinating biology—how the pain reflex is intended to work, how our connective tissue holds on to it, and how we can use Essentrics to heal it once and for all.

CHAPTER 2

Our Living Matrix of Tissue—and How It Can Heal Us

We've all felt many kinds of pain—from cuts and scrapes to headaches to sore muscles. Each of these types of pain emits a unique signal (or set of signals) that is transmitted throughout the body. Yet one of the distinctive things about pain is that it can't be objectively measured—our primary means of studying pain is through our own subjective experience.

This subjectivity of experience has mystified pain researchers for decades, and has made it tremendously difficult to accurately diagnose, let alone cure, pain. But recent groundbreaking studies on the function of our body's connective tissue may hold the answers to why we all have such varied experiences of pain—and how we can heal it.

Pain Follows Many Paths

One thing we do know: Pain is *experienced* through the nervous system. Our peripheral nerves stretch from the spinal cord to the muscles, bones, joints, organs, and skin. On the very end of our nerve fibers are a specific type of receptors, called nociceptors, which make up an early-warning system that sounds the alarm when we experience tissue damage—or even when we experience *potential* tissue damage.

When the nociceptors sense something that could cause harm—such as the hot stove that your hand just brushed—they send electrical impulses along your peripheral nerves to your spinal cord and brain. Those nerves release neurotransmitters that communicate the pain message farther along the channel, all the way up to the thalamus in your brain.

Once the message arrives, the thalamus—an oval mass of gray matter in the middle of the brain—then passes it along to three other areas of your brain:

The somatosensory cortex, which tells you where and how intensely you feel the pain.

The limbic system, which tells you how you experience the pain emotionally.

The frontal cortex, which tells you how to process the pain intellectually.

In each of these areas, the pain message is specific to the individual experiencing it. Depending on your body's unique release of neurotransmitters and your current state of health—including preexisting injuries and baseline inflammation levels—the pain message might be amplified or quieted down at any point in the communication chain. Other variables, too, influence how you experience the pain message, including your current emotional state, memories of pain you've experienced in the past, or your determination to "grin and bear it." All of these mental and emotional messages can influence the way you feel pain—and they all can happen simultaneously, in a split second.

In the case of chronic pain, pain messages that were once simple can get stuck in a rut. Like a needle caught in a groove of a vinyl album, pain messages can start skipping and replaying endlessly in a "pain loop." Instead of heading in a singular direction—from nociceptors to peripheral nerves to spinal cord to brain—these pain messages hit the spinal cord and then the neurotransmitters just explode, branching off in all directions at once. One of their targets is glial cells.

Making up most of the brain's connective tissue, glial cells were originally presumed to function like nervous system putty—*glia* comes from the Greek word for "glue." For decades, scientists thought glial cells were simple structures that held together the higher-functioning elements of the nervous system. But new research has revealed that glial cells are incredibly active in almost every aspect of nervous system function, including:

Brain development

Homeostasis

Information processing, learning, and memory

Formation of myelin (the protective sheaths around nerves)

Regeneration of certain neurons

Glial cells, it turns out, play a key role in how we experience our senses—and our pain. They can lessen our pain, make it worse, or even distort it completely. Once glial cells are activated by the original neurotransmitter release, their DNA synthesizes new proteins, which spill out of the cell membranes and interact with other glial cells around them. Depending on the message being transmitted, those other cells may then release their own neurotransmitters, whose DNA synthesizes their own proteins and spill out again. As this chain continues, the pain loop is reinforced, becoming stronger and more distorted. The original pain signal becomes just a tiny part of what you experience—instead, each time the pain loop is triggered, you're also feeling the echoes of past pain messages, which can get stronger and stronger, depending on the degree of feedback.

In a TED talk from March 2011, Dr. Elliot Krane, a professor of anesthesiology at Stanford Medical School, described this pain feedback loop and likened it to the work of a rogue electrician who has sneaked into your house and rewired all of your circuits so that the next time you flip a light switch, your toilet flushes or your computer turns on. The rewiring completely distorts the subjective experience of pain and may leave it quite far from the original source of the pain. At this point, the distortion becomes a disease in itself: the scourge of chronic pain.[1]

Chronic pain can be incredibly tenacious, and it becomes more entrenched with every trigger. This chain reaction is part of what makes healing from pain so difficult—and why pain medications are woefully inadequate and unequal to the task. Certain pain relievers might temporarily mute the pain signals, and others might tamp down the inflammation so that the body is not as primed for pain—but unless you can reprogram the pain transmission itself, you cannot disrupt the pain loop.

Is it possible to reprogram the transmission? Possible, but challenging. Unfortunately, we can't just send in a little scavenger to scoop up all the misfiring glial cells and get rid of our rogue electrician. Some researchers, like Dr. Krane, are investigating drugs that can be used to target the glial cells directly. But what seems to be most effective is to use nature's own remedy, which turns out to be a more basic, mechanical, and long-term solution: gentle exercise.

HOW ARE INFLAMMATION AND PAIN LINKED?

The most commonly used pain relievers actually don't directly target pain itself—instead, they target inflammation. Nonsteroidal anti-inflammatory drugs (NSAIDs), such as ibuprofen, acetaminophen, and even the humble aspirin, try to stop the inflammatory cascade from even starting. Inflammation is triggered when the body is trying to fight something—bacteria, viruses, injury, or, in the case of autoimmunity, our own body tissues. To fight the foreign substances, the body releases white blood cells, which increase blood flow and swelling in the affected area. But while this is meant as a protective process, the resulting swelling and excess inflammatory substances can irritate the nerves, exacerbate pressure on the joints, and lead to serious damage.

Exercise is one way we can attempt to communicate with the misfit cells and persuade them to stand down and stop transmitting (and duplicating) all those extra pain messages. That could be because exercise can *directly* manipulate glial cells' connective tissue cousins—the sheets and bands of fascia that move and stretch throughout the body.

Connective Tissue: The Missing Link

As we've discussed, until recently scientists viewed the musculoskeletal system as a workhorse—responsible for posture and movement, and not much else. But a new field of research is finally helping to prove what has long been understood by practitioners in disciplines like traditional Chinese medicine and physical therapy: that the musculoskeletal system has a wide-ranging influence on all bodily systems.

In a line of research that spans more than twenty years, pioneering researcher Dr. Helene Langevin has suggested that our fascia functions as a "living matrix." Her research offers evidence that this connective tissue is in a constant state of communication—with itself, with other parts of the body, and with the outside world—helping coordinate and regulate the activities of many major bodily systems. As Dr. Langevin stated in her groundbreaking 2006 paper in the journal *Medical Hypotheses*, "Since connective tissue is intimately associated with all other tissues (e.g., lungs, intestine), connective tissue signaling may coherently influence (and be influenced by) the normal or pathological function of a wide variety of organ systems."

Dr. Langevin described the wide-ranging role of connective tissue in *The Scientist* in 2013:

[Connective tissue] joins your thigh to your calf; your hand to your arm; your breastbone to your clavicle. As you move, it allows your muscles to glide past one another. It acts like a net suspending your organs and a high-tech adhesive holding your cells in place while relaying messages between them. Connective tissue is one of the most integral components of the human machine. Indeed, one could draw a line between any two points of the body via a path of connective tissue. This network is so extensive and ubiquitous that if we were to lose every organ, muscle, bone, nerve, and blood vessel in our bodies, we would still maintain the same shape: our "connective-tissue body."[2]

Thankfully, after decades of neglect, more researchers—including those interested in the therapeutic applications of exercise programs like Essentrics—are focused on exploring the healing potential of our connective tissue. The hope is that we can discover new ways to silence the ever-present signaling of chronic pain and get back to living full, pain-free lives.

The Function of Fascia

When you look at most anatomy books, you'll see drawings of bones and ligaments, tendons and muscles, but you'll rarely see the whitish or semi-translucent bands and sheets that are involved in most muscular movements—the fascia (or, to use the plural, the fasciae). Fascia has traditionally been known as an uninterrupted, three-dimensional web that surrounds and interpenetrates muscles, groups of muscles, blood vessels, and nerves, binding some structures together while permitting others to slide smoothly over each other.[3] However, researchers are now debating new theories about the function of our fascia.

The existence of these tight-fitting lubricated sleeves enables the nerves, muscles, and all other human tissue to stretch or shrink as we move, and then return to their original shape with total ease. These sleeves are one reason why we maintain our shape as we reach, bend, crunch, and extend our body throughout the passage of a day.

You've probably never given a second thought as to why your body looks the same in the evening as it did in the morning. Since moving creates a kneading action on our soft tissue, we could easily change shape every day—but we don't! Why is that? The fasciae encase all our tissues, giving them a limited, lubricated area in which to move. And as we stretch or contract our muscles continuously, the fasciae allow those movements—indeed, they love them!—but always return to their original starting shape.

When we raise an arm, the muscle cells must slide to permit the lengthening of a muscle; the nerves embedded within the muscles must also be able to slide, and the tendons must slide back within their sheaths. This intricate dance occurs each time we do something as simple as throwing a ball to a dog or waving hello to a friend.

Also essential to movement is the fluid within the fascia, which is actually liquid, or "gel-like" connective tissue. (I referred to this in my first book as the body's "oily bath.") This liquid nourishes our tissue and prevents its various components from adhering to one another; without this critical lubrication, our cells become glued together, making us feel stiff.

Immobility is one of the most common causes of pain because it leads to the solidifying or hardening of this liquid connective tissue. Every time we move, we create a subtle pumping motion that gently pushes fluid through our living matrix. Immobility permits the fluid to congeal; as it does so, the tissue layers become somewhat sticky. That's why when our movement is restricted over a prolonged period—such as when we recover from a surgery or an injury—we start to feel very stiff and sore.

If connective tissue is the integrating matrix for the whole body, you can see how congested and glued tissues might start to become a serious issue. What kinds of terrible biological missteps might develop if we had massive logjams of adhesion right in the middle of our fasciae? You've likely heard the saying massage therapists often use: "You've got issues in your tissues." Until we release those knots and blocks in our fasciae, we may be preventing all kinds of critical physiological communication from getting through.

Dr. Langevin's research clearly shows that our connective tissue relays different types of messages, including electrical, cellular, and tissue remodeling signals. Each of these signals then creates patterns that interact with one another and evolve over time. By this theory, if there is a blockage in our connective tissue, pain messages could be magnified in loops, tissue repair messages could be blocked, and even signals of pleasure or relaxation might be hampered or blunted.

Just imagine how much better we could all feel if our bodies had none of those blockages—and our connective tissue was able to facilitate open and direct communication with all of our major organs. The good news is, that's entirely possible. These messages can be manipulated by simple changes in our movements and posture.

Given the emerging science of connective tissue and what I've learned from helping people suffering from chronic pain, I know the Essentrics program works to improve the natural integrity and healing power of connective tissue—thereby improving all the communication that's taking place, moment by moment, within our living matrix.

CHAPTER 3

When the Matrix Gets Disrupted

Many common causes of pain stem from neither diseases nor injuries, making them nearly impossible to diagnose. Doctors have a hard time finding a label for this kind of pain because there is nothing clinically wrong with the patient—other than the subjective experience of pain—nor are they able to offer any relief aside from surgery or medication.

While Essentrics cannot solve every case of chronic pain, I have seen it help many of these mystery cases. In this chapter, I take a closer look at the sources of chronic pain that are the result of unbalanced and immobile muscles along with atrophy and hardening of connective tissues. The fastest way to fix these problems is to simply reverse what caused them in the first place—either the wrong type of movement or no movement at all.

When it comes to exercise, we need to start thinking like Goldilocks: not too little, not too much, but just right. Doing just-right exercises can rebalance muscle groups, improve alignment, break up adhesions, help blood and oxygen flow freely, and—finally, permanently—heal your pain.

Our Sedentary Lifestyle: The #1 Cause of Pain

D r. James Levine, director of the initiative Obesity Solutions at the Mayo Clinic at Arizona State University, coined the saying "Sitting is the new smoking." The statement may seem provocative, but it is absolutely accurate. Immobility is a silent killer, one of the most damaging lifestyle choices we can make. Being sedentary slows or even stops certain vital bodily processes: Our circulation slows. Our arteries start collecting deposits. Our lymphatic system doesn't get flushed out. Our cells become less sensitive to insulin and our pancreas weakens. Our muscles atrophy, their cells starting to die off.

By not moving, we've given our body the signal that it's no longer necessary—so our body literally begins to prepare for death.

Immobility is as dangerous as a car crash or a major accident, yet it is far less obvious. It causes its devastation when we are doing absolutely nothing. A sedentary lifestyle has been linked to the following medical conditions and diseases:

- Arthritis
- Autoimmune conditions
- Cancer
- Depression
- Early-onset dementia
- Erectile dysfunction
- Heart disease
- Muscle atrophy
- Obesity
- Premature aging
- Sleep disorders
- Type 2 diabetes

Being sedentary clearly causes damage to our organs. So how do we define "sedentary"? The answer may surprise you. Being sedentary is defined as sitting for longer than six hours a day—a passive activity that anyone with an office job is typically required to do at least five days a week. Many of us who sit long hours at a computer may mistakenly believe that if we work out in the morning or evening, we'll be inoculated against the effects of so much sitting. Not true!

In 2003, the *Journal of the American Medical Association* published a landmark study quantifying the effects of sedentary behavior. In analysis of the lifestyle habits of over fifty thousand women, the researchers found that every two-hour increment of time spent sitting (in this case, watching TV) per day was associated with a 23 percent increase in obesity and a 14 percent increase in the risk of diabetes.[1] Given that our time spent staring at screens has only increased over the past decade, these risks would naturally seem to be compounding.

Indeed, in January 2015, the *Annals of Internal Medicine* published a meta-analysis showing that more than half of an average person's life is spent sitting: in a car, on a bus, at work, in front of the TV, or at the dinner table. The Canadian researchers reviewed forty-seven studies that assessed the health effects of a sedentary lifestyle on thousands of people. They found that people who sat for prolonged periods had a higher risk dying from a multitude of illnesses as compared with their more active peers. What was particularly upsetting about this study was the finding that, even when people exercised for an hour a day, if they sat for 50 percent of their life, they were still at risk from the effects of the "sitting disease."[2]

I consider myself a very active person because I do 30 to 60 minutes of exercise a day, park as far away as possible and walk to my destination, use the stairs when it is realistic, and go for walks when I have time. However, I spend many more hours writing, correcting exams, working on projects, traveling, and meeting with colleagues. As I do all these things, I sit. In fact, as I sit to write this book, I am surrounded by an office full of people sitting at their computers, whether designing workouts or editing TV shows.

When I was working on my first book, *Aging Backwards*, the research on atrophy scared the living daylights out of me. As soon as I understood the dangers of permitting one's muscle cells to atrophy from lack of use, I rapidly became my own best student. I've rarely missed a day since to exercise each of my 650 muscles. I've always enjoyed exercise, but now I'm even more aware that if you don't use it, you *will* lose it! When I do have to sit at my desk for hours at a time, I try to get up and move for a few minutes every half hour or so, which research shows does help to counteract the negative effects of sitting.

In today's working world, there seems to be no avoiding being sedentary, which is why we need to navigate ourselves through this dangerous new reality and find healthy and sustainable solutions. Doing nothing may seem harmless, but we have to remind ourselves that the human body was designed to move. Movement is at the root of all life; it's what keeps the engines of every one of our trillions of cells alive. When we stop moving, we start dying one cell at a time!

What Happens When We *Don't* Move

The question of why immobility creates so much havoc in our bodies is answered in our cells. Our life force is contained in our trillions of cells. They require constant motion partly so that they don't become glued to each other, so that nutrient-rich blood can circulate to every cell. When we are immobile, the cells stick to one another. A gluing chain reaction takes place with the neighboring cells, until large sheets of glued-together connective tissue harden around our organs and muscles, further immobilizing us. And embedded in this hardened tissue are even more dying, atrophying cells.

At first we experience a sensation of stiffness—but as the immobility accelerates, the stiffness increases. Immobilized muscle cells slowly atrophy and shrink, in time squeezing the joints together. This squeezing damages the joints, leading to chronic pain and, if not reversed, the need for surgery or even joint replacement.

Our cells require both nourishment and cleansing for survival; these tasks are carried out by the circulatory system. The circulatory system is designed to deliver nutrients and remove toxins by delivering fresh supplies of blood and oxygen around the body. With sedentary behavior, our circulation slows to a crawl, and very little nourishment is delivered to our cells. When a cell is starved of nutrients and has no way of releasing stored toxins, it suffocates from within. Basically, when we are sedentary, the body cannot use its natural, self-healing powers.

Immobility leaves us feeling tired and unwell, and makes recovery slow and incomplete—and, if we wait too long, more and more difficult. As I talked about in my first book, *Aging Backwards*, the negative feedback cycle of sedentary behavior can quickly get out of hand. Cell loss or atrophy triggered by immobility makes controlling weight extremely difficult because we sacrifice our mitochondria, the calorie-burning furnaces tucked into every cell. Obesity quickly becomes another self-perpetuating loop, with fat cells proliferating, muscle cells atrophying, and our body becoming weaker, flabbier, and stiffer over time.

Pain Is Unresolved Stiffness

When we wake up in the morning, we usually feel a little stiff from a long night of immobility. The less we move upon waking, the stiffer we feel—but after some stretching, the stiffness can go away.

Magnify that just-out-of-bed stiffness many times over, and you may better understand the sort of stiffness that many people chalk up to the aging process. Most people respond to this discomfort by moving less. But the less we move, the more our connective tissue solidifies, creating a chain reaction and exacerbating the problem. Remember: Pain is a message from the brain telling us that there is something dangerous happening to our body. The message of stiffness is a *precursor* to the pain message.

When any part of the body is immobilized, whether through surgery, injury, or lifestyle, the liquid connective tissue starts to congeal and harden. Over time, this liquid connective tissue gets gooey and harder, causing muscles to shrink from inactivity. A chain reaction takes over, aging us rapidly and painfully. And if we don't rid ourselves of the stiffness—which can be quite easily done through a short, gentle full-body workout—we will likely soon experience pain. To stop stiffness from spiraling into pain, we must stretch out the stiffness, which nourishes our cells and lubricates our living matrix.

The congealing of connective tissue doesn't happen uniformly around the body. As we walk, we may favor one hip over the other without realizing it. If we routinely lean on one elbow, the ribs on the opposite side might become glued together, leading to an imbalance in the musculoskeletal system.

Whether you are thin or overweight, weak muscles will deform the alignment of any joint, from the feet and ankles up through the hips into the spine. In addition to all the perils mentioned earlier, a sedentary lifestyle usually involves not only slouching but also not engaging all of our muscles and walking with a heavy footstep, slamming our feet down as we step. Heavy walking slowly breaks down the surface of the joints, damaging the knees, ankles, and hips, causing painful joint damage.

The Widespread Consequences of Weak Muscles

Our muscular structure is the machinery that moves our body and supports the bones, organs, and all other tissue. Muscles are designed to be strong enough to allow our body to feel weightless as we move around all day long. When our muscles are well cared for, we forget they exist—our body just does what we want it to do without pain or difficulty. Maybe that's why the muscles are often referred to as the "guardians of our youth."

But when our muscles are weak, we not only feel heavy and chronically tired but also unhealthy overall. Some of the most obvious consequences of weak muscles can be seen in our bones and joints. Weak muscles cannot prevent the weight of the body from compressing and pinching the joints and the connective tissue—leading to extremely painful premature arthritis and joint disease. Weak muscles also cannot protect us from losing precious bone mass, which leads to osteoporosis.

Weak muscles also endanger the health of our cardiovascular system. The vascular system—a network of sixty-nine thousand miles of veins, arteries, and capillaries that deliver blood throughout the body—requires strong skeletal muscles to keep things moving. Muscle movement creates a pumping action that naturally assists the circulation of blood throughout the entire body. Inactive, weak muscles, by default, leave the job of circulating the blood to the cardiac muscle. While the role of the vascular system is to circulate, the role of the cardiac muscle is to pump—so without the assistance of strong skeletal muscles, the cardiac muscle ends up doing double duty.

Digestion is also affected by weak muscles. When abdominal muscles are weak, the intestines have nothing to push against. This makes elimination slow and uncomfortable. When the torso muscles are weak, the lower body sinks backward while the upper body slouches; this poor posture crushes the esophagus, making swallowing painful and leading to acid reflux.

These are just a few of the reasons why weak muscles can lead to chronic pain. Muscles are designed to be strong, not weak. They strengthen rapidly with even the easiest exercises. The smallest increase in strength will rapidly improve our ability to move easily. The most important aspect of muscles is that they are designed to move the full body; it is by doing full-body movement that the magic of pain relief and improved health takes place.

Imbalanced Muscles

Having imbalanced muscles may sound like a relatively harmless problem—yet that is very far from the truth. Muscular imbalances are one of the key triggers that set off the chain reaction throughout the body that causes serious damage to joints and muscles. Consider that two of the worst pain conditions caused by imbalances in the skeletal muscles are back pain and arthritis. The amazing truth is that rebalancing the muscles is relatively easy with the correct exercises.

Treating back pain is a billion-dollar industry, draining both public and private purses. Lost wages for the employee and lost productivity for the employer make chronic back pain a costly condition. Beyond the issue of cost, chronic back pain can be so overpowering that any relief is welcome, even when that relief is fleeting and accompanied by serious risks and side effects. That's why thousands of people turn to pain relievers or undergo back surgery every year—despite the fact that pain relievers have only temporary effects.

Recently, however, some doctors have recognized an alternative to surgery and drugs. According to Dr. Hamilton Hall, the founder of the Canadian Back Institute (now CBI Health Group) and the author of *The Back Doctor*, 80 percent of back pain can be relieved with correct rebalancing exercises. Thousands of people undergo back surgery every year—and it doesn't always work. In many cases, correct exercises are not only cheaper and less painful than surgery—they are what's actually needed. Preventing and adjusting muscular imbalance is the foundation of lasting back pain relief.

To better understand the role of muscular imbalance in back pain, it helps to understand the role muscles play in keeping joints balanced. The thirty-three vertebrae of the spine are designed to move in many directions: forward, back, side to side, and diagonally. Directly or indirectly attached to the spine are dozens of muscles whose job it is to move the spine in all its many directions. Some muscles help us twist, others help us bend forward, and still others bend us backward.

When the spine is poorly aligned, a group of back muscles will become overworked when it tries to pull the vertebrae back into alignment. When the overworked group can no longer sustain the constant state of stress, it goes into spasm. Anyone who has ever experienced a back spasm knows that the pain is excruciating and intolerable! Rebalancing the full musculature of the spine helps realign the full spinal vertebrae, taking the constant stress off the overworked muscles.

This is why having good posture and a fully mobile torso is essential in preventing back pain. Anytime our spine is not in correct alignment, we will inevitably suffer from back, shoulder, or neck pain. Having poor posture, slouching, or sitting at a desk all day tends to weaken the spinal muscles and thus leads to chronic back pain. We hear about bulging, herniated, or slipped discs, or disc decay or arthritis—the root cause of many of these excruciating back problems can be traced to imbalanced muscles.

MY EXPERIENCE WITH BACK PAIN

My ballet training led me to have poor alignment in both of my femurs (thighbones). This alignment is taught to ballerinas as "good" alignment, but it forces the thigh muscles to exist in a constant state of tension. I thought that tension meant my muscles were strong, which they were, but when a muscle is contracted it shortens, along with the surrounding muscles. So for me, the constant tension didn't stay in the thigh muscles but spiraled into a related group called the psoas muscles, which attach to the lower spine.

By the time I reached forty, the contracted psoas muscles had pulled my L4 and L5 vertebrae (the lowest two vertebrae in the lumbar part of the spine) out of alignment, creating a bulging disc and premature arthritis of the spine. I was in a lot of pain for a long time. That's when I met Dr. Bradley Bosick, a chiropractor and neurologist in Denver, Colorado, who explained to me that muscles should never be in a permanent state of contraction. Healthy muscles are meant to alternate between relaxation and contraction continuously throughout the day. Anytime anything is in a constant state of contraction, it is vulnerable to damage.

A slight shift in the alignment of my femurs instantly relieved the tension in my thigh and psoas muscles—and the muscles relaxed. That was when I finally understood the root cause of my chronic back pain: poor alignment unbalancing my thigh and back muscles.

Bad posture habits like mine are slow to change, because the correct posture feels unnatural and wrong at first. It took me a while to realign my thighbones and rebalance my muscles, but the difference in comfort, ease, and energy I've experienced since then is truly amazing.

Creating Essentrics helped me rebalance my spine and get rid of back pain. I have remained pain-free ever since—unless I miss too many days of exercise. Learning how to stand correctly has also de-stressed my thigh muscles, releasing what was once a constant tension on my spine.

Joint Imbalance

The human body has 384 joints. Joints are movable body parts in which adjacent bones are held together by a complex system of muscles, tendons, and ligaments. At the head of each bone is a lubricated, glassy surface that permits joints to glide effortlessly as we move. Joint damage is often caused when muscles shrink or shorten around the joint, squeezing the joints so tightly together that the lubrication required to make them slide can't get into the joint. With no lubrication, the glassy surface is no longer slippery, and becomes drier and drier. Every movement, from standing to sitting, acts like sandpaper to grind away the protective glassy surface until the bones begin to grind. This is excruciatingly painful! We have to keep our joints well aligned, and the muscles surrounding them well balanced, to prevent them from being damaged or injured. Most joint imbalance begins in the muscles.

As noted earlier, our spine has thirty-three vertebrae. Vertebrae are designed to comfortably permit the torso to bend forward as we pick something up, bend sideways as we get out of a car, and twist as we turn to look behind us. Our fingers and knees, in contrast, have joints like hinges of a door—we don't want our fingers or knees to be capable of moving in the same circular motion as our spine. Walking would be very unstable if our knees were capable of circular mobility, and holding objects would be awkward if our fingers moved all over the place! This is why muscles are designed to protect and maintain the alignment and range of motion of each specific joint. When the muscles surrounding any joint become imbalanced, the joint will lose its safe alignment and inevitably suffer damage. Pain is the message that tells us when that damage is happening.

Arthritis is a common result of muscle imbalance that leads to joint damage, and it can affect every joint of the body. The definition of a well-balanced muscle is that it must be equally strong and flexible and capable of easily doing the job it is designed for. When we don't use our muscles over the years, they weaken, shrink, and can no longer support our body easily. Instead of being supported by our muscles, the weight of our body settles heavily into our spine, hips, knees, and ankles. The impact of gravity and our weight slowly wears away at all the protective cushions in our joints until the joint heads are exposed, their surfaces begin to grind, and inflammation results. This is known as arthritis. Arthritis pain feels like a knife shooting through the body—not a pleasant experience and something we should all try to avoid.

Arthritis takes decades to damage the joints. It doesn't happen overnight! During those years, correct exercise can prevent or reverse much of the damage. Without such exercise, there will come a point of no return, when joint replacement or spinal surgery is necessary. The only way to slow down arthritis is to simultaneously stretch and strengthen the atrophying muscles through regular, gentle exercise.

On the other hand, it is very common for serious athletes and gym rats alike to over-train their muscles to the point of limited mobility within the muscle fibers. Muscle fibers are designed to have a great deal of flexibility, like an old-fashioned telescope—they should be able to go from contracted (shortened) to lengthened by up to one hundred times in a nanosecond. An overtrained muscle stays contracted and firm to the touch, day and night, and can barely release to ten times its potential length. When the muscle never has an opportunity to stretch out to its full potential, an excessive tension builds within its fibers. The brain identifies the unreleased tension as pain, which is what people in gyms usually feel after a hard workout. Unchecked, the constant tension will lead to serious damage. If the training has been excessive some of the pain will also be due to inflammation. The brain, which wants us to be healthy, is warning us in the only way it can—through a pain message. Unaddressed pain from unbalanced muscle fibers goes on to cause serious damage to our joints.

Chronic Knee Pain

Knee pain is very common and often caused by muscular imbalance, poor bone alignment, or both. The knee joint moves like a door hinge, permitting the bones to swing forward and back. If a door hinge is loose, the door will swing unstably, causing damage to the full frame. The knee hinge works exactly the same—when the knee hinge is off balance, it causes damage not only to the actual knee joint but also to the entire body's structural frame.

Most of us walk with our weight rolling toward either the inside of our leg or the outside (eversion and inversion, respectively). To figure out which imbalance you have, take a look at the soles your shoes to see which side of the heels wear out. If your feet are everting or inverting, which most people's do, you are prone to knee or hip pain.

The full leg muscles on the side you roll toward will have to do more work than those on the other side. One side of your leg will get tighter, and the opposite side will get weaker. In time, this muscular imbalance will pull the leg bones out of alignment. Every time you walk, the weight of your body will no longer be cleanly distributed through the center of the leg and knee but will instead sink to one side. This poor alignment of the bones will lead to joint damage—and a whole slew of potential knee conditions can arise, from arthritis to sciatica. And, boy, will you feel this as knee pain! Heed the pain's warning, and do something about it.

When you correct the imbalance through full-body stretching and strengthening, the pressure or squeezing together of the joints disappears. Unfortunately, the resulting cartilage damage cannot be self-healed—whatever has been destroyed will stay destroyed—but when we stretch and strengthen the muscles around the knee, we can prevent further damage from occurring.

Arthritis is a condition of progressive degrees. When caught early enough, it can be controlled so that you will never experience pain. Depending on the degree of damage, each person experiences a different degree of pain relief, and many people feel total pain relief when they do their exercises daily.

Hip Pain

The causes of hip pain are multiple: falls and other injuries, arthritis, torn labra (the rims of soft tissue around the hip sockets), and muscle imbalances. Exercises similar to those suggested for knee pain generally address the wide range of hip problems.

Paradoxically, the most common sufferers of hip pain come from two opposite demographic groups: sedentary middle-aged folks or really active people. However, the pain and immobility from which they both end up suffering is similar.

Muscles are designed to support the skeleton, and that includes our joints and bones. With regard to the first group, as noted earlier in this chapter, a sedentary lifestyle leads to weak muscles. Weak muscles cannot prevent the body's weight from slamming into the hip joint with every step we make. This causes joint damage in the hip just as it does in the knee. With regard to the second group, athletes, professional and amateur, usually slam their hip joints together with every movement, whether it's running, diving, hitting, landing, or punching. Athletes generally have little awareness of the damage that repetitive impact causes their joints, and they tend to have very high rates of hip replacement surgery.

The degeneration of the hip joints takes place over years, enabling us to become accustomed to feeling stiff and being weak. We chalk it up to aging. Eventually, the stiffness turns to mild pain. As the pain gets stronger, we visit our doctor, who may tell us that in the distant future we will need a hip replacement. The suggestion of a future hip replacement is accompanied by the explanation that, before the doctor can operate, we have to wait until the pain is unbearable and the joint totally destroyed. Much of this is referred to as hip arthritis.

As with the knees, imbalanced muscles in the hip are often caused by an incorrect stance of the feet, leading to poor alignment of the leg bones. If we roll in or roll out on our ankles, we pull the knees in or outward. This leads to a chain reaction of imbalance throughout the skeletal structure, from the soles of our feet through our ankles, knees, and hips. This imbalance will force one group of hip muscles to work harder than the other. As one group works harder, it naturally becomes stronger, while the other group becomes weaker and shrinks. This imbalance eventually leads to joint damage. The hip exercises in part 2 are designed to rebalance these muscles and reverse any pressure on the hip.

JUST FOR SENIORS: HIP PAIN

When seniors remain sedentary, they accelerate their aging process by permitting their muscles to rapidly atrophy and weaken. Many sedentary seniors have insufficient strength to support their skeleton. This causes their joints to slam heavily together, making all movement painful. Many types of seniors' hip pain, including sciatica and arthritis, is caused by weakness. Walking upstairs can become problematic when hip and leg muscles are too weak to lift the weight of the body. The good news is that even a small amount of exercise will rapidly strengthen seniors' muscles and thereby relieve the pain. After all, muscles are created to be strong, and that includes seniors' muscles!

Poor Alignment

I like to explain the difference between good alignment (which is also called clean alignment) and poor alignment with a housebuilding analogy. If we hire a team of five workers to build one house and a team of ten workers to build an equivalent house, and ask both teams to finish the work in the same amount of time, common sense tells us that after finishing the house the five workers would be more exhausted than the ten workers. Well, good alignment is like using all ten muscles of a joint to move us around instead of five muscles—it's more efficient, less tiring, and causes less damage over the long term.

The weight of the body must flow all the way through the skeleton's bones, finishing in the soles of the feet. However, good alignment starts with the feet and flows upward to the head, not the reverse. If our normal stance has our feet rolling outward, it will distort the alignment of our leg bones. The distortion will be forced to continue up the legs, twisting the knees, hips, and spine. In other words, when our feet are in poor alignment, all the bones in our body above our feet will then become poorly aligned.

While good alignment begins at the feet, moving upward, our weight distribution starts at our head and flows downward through the skeleton. If we have good alignment, there will be no stress on the joints. In addition, our muscles will be functioning in perfect balance.

Not so if we have poor alignment. With poor alignment the weight of the body will flow unevenly from the head to the toes, overstressing some muscles and leading to joint damage.

We have twenty-six bones in our feet; the joints between them need to be correctly aligned. Any joint that is incorrectly aligned will place the adjoining joints and muscles in a state of permanent imbalance and stress. Over a lifetime of poor foot alignment, the damage will spiral itself up our legs and manifest itself as ankle, knee, hip, and back pain.

Even though the feet play the initial and decidedly most important role in establishing clean alignment, they are by no means the only parts of our bodies that need attention. To understand alignment, you have to look at the full skeleton. Any joint that is out of alignment will lead to instability, stressed muscles, and pain. A clean alignment, one that includes fingers to toes and every joint in between, ensures that all the surrounding muscles are firing at their maximum effectiveness. Clean alignment means that the neurological loops from the brain to the muscles and from the brain to the organs will be clear and efficient. These loops are essential to keep the immune system strong and our body healthy and energetic. Clean alignment permits the joints to glide smoothly and safely, free from potential damage like arthritis. If we maintain clean alignment, there's no reason our joints can't remain vital and strong well into our golden years.

Posture

You have good posture when all of your muscles are as strong as they are flexible. Good posture should reflect a relaxed mobility. To me, poor posture looks like the Tin Man, upright but stiff and uncomfortable. Good posture should be easier to support than poor posture, no matter if you're sitting or standing! In my view, the definition of good posture is a state of perfect alignment in which our 384 joints are perfectly aligned and our 650 muscles shift continuously from tension to relaxation.

Few people have that type of good posture holding their torso upright and their chest open with full relaxed mobility. Many people appear to have good posture, but they are in fact very stiff and rigid. Often their upper back is slightly rounded while their lower back is tight. Rounded backs are usually a sign of overbuilt pectorals and trapezius muscles (chest muscles). Tight hips are a sign of tight gluteus muscles (tight bum). Overbuilt or tight muscles are in constant stress—and we know that when muscles are in a constant state of stress, injuries and pain result.

Poor posture unbalances the erector spinae (muscles that keep the back straight), placing stress on the spinal vertebrae. If your teeth are crooked, an orthodontist uses braces to deliberately put stress on them to pull them into correct alignment with your jaw. But when your erector spinae are imbalanced, they pull one or more vertebrae out of alignment with the rest of the spine, causing slipped or bulging discs.

You can see now why unbalanced muscles are directly related to conditions such as bulging, herniated, or slipped discs; arthritis of the spine; and the need for spinal surgery. It's a chicken-and-egg situation: correct alignment helps keep the muscles balanced correctly, while well-balanced muscles help keep the spine well aligned.

THE FALLACY OF BALLET DANCERS' "PERFECT" POSTURE

When you think of someone with perfect posture, you might think of a prima ballerina, right? Unfortunately, this is a common misperception. As a ballet dancer, I used to *look* like I had excellent posture—my spine was upright and my shoulders open. However, at the time I was forcing my spine out of its natural *S* curve into a straight line.

A healthy spine has a natural double-*S* curve. Ballet dancers must be able to stand en pointe and pirouette without falling over. To do this, they are trained from childhood to line up their bones in as straight a line as possible, from head to toe. This forces the dancers to tuck in their tailbone so their bums don't stick out, to avoid a weight imbalance as they spin. As a result, the natural alignment of most ballet dancers' spines becomes deformed. In my case, the deliberate deformation of my lower spine led to years of debilitating chronic back pain. While I was in pain, my X-rays showed two slipped discs. Through regular, gentle, full-body exercise, I returned my spine to its correct alignment and, with it, became permanently relieved of pain.

People often blame computer use and texting as the major cause of poor posture, but I am not convinced that poor posture is a modern phenomenon. In fact, I believe it's actually encouraged by our anatomical design! Our eyes are in the front of our head, not the back, and when we walk, we do so forward, not backward. When we sit, our knees bend in front of our body, not behind it. From the way I see it, it's normal that we would gradually slump forward if we permit ourselves to. Computers may be compounding the problem, but since the beginning of time, humans have been inclined to have poor posture. After years of permitting the head to hang forward, the muscles and connective tissue of the upper back thicken from semi-immobility.

The image that generally comes to mind when we think of poor posture is an elderly woman stooped over with her neck bowed forward. The forward rounding of the spine, called kyphosis, may be the result of a congenital defect or may be developed later in life as a result of osteoporosis or poor posture. It becomes visible when osteoporosis has reached an advanced stage, forcing the neck and head to fall forward. Non-osteoporosis or congenital forms of kyphosis occur in men and women alike when they assume a rounded-back posture for many years—in other words, when they have consistently poor posture. The ensuing rounding of the spine stress the individual vertebrae at the point where the neck and the spine meet. As the neck droops forward the vertebrae shrink and become thinner. With kyphosis you will find little to no mobility in the person's vertebrae and soft tissue in the upper back. When the spine is in a rounded posture like kyphosis, the muscles are in a constant state of stress, as the poor alignment leads to constant muscle imbalance. This chronic condition can be very painful.

In addition to the damage to the vertebrae, with every inch our neck bows forward, we load ten pounds of stress onto the supporting spine muscles. These muscles are then in a state of tension, and this tension is further increased by the continuous muscle contraction; they never get a moment to relax and release, as healthy muscles must do. Poor posture, with even an inch of forward bowing of the head, is exhausting and painful.

Poor posture actually shrinks our bodies. We don't just give the appearance that we have become smaller—we actually *do* become smaller. This is because poor posture leads to atrophy.

Shrinking or atrophying is painful, just as growing pains were painful when we were adolescents. It does not happen evenly; as we shrink, it occurs unevenly throughout our bodies, creating the vicious cycle of muscular imbalance and joint damage.

The process doesn't happen overnight. It takes years for the bones to weaken and the ligaments, tendons, fasciae, and other forms of connective tissue to atrophy. The good news is you can reverse both the poor posture and the atrophy. Improving your posture isn't rocket science—it just takes persistence. Good posture means pulling your body upward, countering the force of gravity. As we stand erect, our muscles naturally pull us upward. As we slouch, our muscles naturally pull us downward. Good posture gently and naturally keeps us young and pain-free by fighting against the force of gravity.[3]

Reforming your posture means teaching yourself to stand, walk, and sit in positions that place the least amount of strain on supporting vertebrae, muscles, and ligaments.

Remember that if you've trained your muscles to support poor posture for decades, this process of retraining can take some time and patience. In fact, when you first start to correct your posture, proper alignment will most likely feel uncomfortable and unnatural. But stick with it. Eventually, it will feel wonderful and effortless.

CORRECTING POOR POSTURE

It's helpful to exercise in front of a full-length mirror, especially when you're starting a program, so you can self-correct your alignment and posture if you notice yourself slouching. Once you become more familiar with the movements, you can take the mirror away.

Overbuilding Muscles

Overbuilding muscles is a common type of imbalance that occurs in athletes and fitness enthusiasts. Today many extreme workout programs have become the rage—a dangerous-for-the-joints rage! There are at least two main reasons why such programs lead to injuries and pain.

First, when one group of muscles becomes overbuilt, they cause an imbalance. The overbuilt group will overpower the weaker muscles, pulling joints out of alignment. This issue is very common in extreme and repetitive sports, and is one of the major reasons for chronic back, neck, and knee pain in these types of training fads.

Second, a healthy, balanced muscle fiber should move like an old-fashioned telescope: it should slide in and out as it contracts and stretches, and it should be capable of stretching and returning to its original shape. Overbuilt muscles are stuck in the contracted phase and have little ability to stretch. Remember that muscles are designed to be equally strong and flexible. There is not a single muscle that is designed to be only contracted to its maximum with limited mobility—not one! Yet this type of muscle training—called *concentric training*—is the basis of almost every sport and fitness method. This is why there are so many injuries and so much pain in sports and fitness.

Ballet is the only technique in the body-training world that builds muscles to be equally flexible and strong. It uses a technique called *eccentric training*, which simultaneously strengthens and stretches muscle fibers. I adopted eccentric training as the basis of Essentrics, because I saw that it protected the joints while maintaining the essence of full mobility within a muscle fiber.

When we analyze the physiology of a muscle cell, it is clear that the protein filaments—thick myosin filaments and thin actin filaments—are designed to slide in and out like a piston. The purpose of a muscle cell is to move—not to be glued in one contracted position. Overbuilding the muscles forces the cells to become locked into a contracted tight position, from which the cells cannot rebound to their original position. In an overbuilt body, the muscles are so tight that they will stay permanently in the same cut, ripped form day and night. That is not healthy or natural. We've been programmed to see excessively contracted muscles as sexy and strong, but what we are actually looking at is muscular imbalance and something that is unhealthy. The prioritization of strength over mobility reduces the range of motion, making movement limited, painful, and prone to injury.

Ironically, the pain from which most athletes suffer is unnecessary; it could be rapidly reduced simply by adding dynamic flexibility to the strength-training regimen. I know this because I have worked with hundreds of professional athletes with the objective of reducing their pain while making them winners! Overbuilding muscles is the major reason why the careers of so many high-performance athletes are cut short prematurely.

But it's not just professional athletes who are suffering—it is everyday people just trying to stay in shape. Even though all evidence suggests that extreme strength training ages the muscles, joints, bones, and immune system, humans are competitive by nature. As they eagerly throw their full heart into a rapid but brutal CrossFit session, even smart, educated people are consciously playing a version of Russian roulette.

I have my theories on why there's such reluctance to acknowledge this issue in sports and athletic training. First, until Essentrics came along, there was no alternative method of effective muscle strengthening. Basically, if you wanted to strengthen your muscles, you had no choice but to overbuild and unbalance them. The second reason is economic. Extreme training is a multibillion-dollar business—there's not much financial incentive for trainers and coaches to discourage their clients from participating in these types of programs.

Scar Tissue Imbalance

Human tissue is like living cloth that has been tightly woven in patterns that permit it to stretch and rebound instantly to its original shape. When we have a scar, from injury or surgery, movement on either side of the scar is blocked. A scar does to the human body what a dam does to the landscape surrounding it. When we construct a dam on a river, it diverts the flow from its natural path, and the land that was previously watered by the river will suffer from drought. Any degree of blockage leads to immobility, which we know is bad for the mechanics of the body and leads to pain. Unfortunately, when we have an operation, scars are inevitable.

To understand the natural flow of human tissue, we can watch the skin of our tummy expand and contract as we breathe deeply in and out. Along with our skin, our muscles, ligaments, tendons, blood, lymph fluids, and nerves also move with every inhalation and exhalation. When we reach above our head to put on a sweater or bend forward to tie a shoe, all the tissues of our body stretch to let us move and then rebound to return to their original shape. When we have a scar, this natural flow is blocked.

That blockage of movement and energy initiates a negative chain reaction that can result in atrophy and imbalance; one side of the scar can look as shriveled as the land on the side of the dam that no longer has access to water. The mobility of both sides of the scarred area is affected.

If the muscles on either side of the scar are not equally stretched and strengthened and returned to normal health, soon they will be starved of nourishment and atrophy. I've seen this happen to many people who have had surgery—from breast or pancreatic cancer surgery to shoulder or back surgery. When people don't spend enough time in physical therapy rehabilitating their scarred areas, the damage will escalate over the years and lead to serious pain.

A scar, even a relatively new one, needs to be stretched and/or massaged in order to prevent damage from atrophy. However, new scars must be treated carefully and differently from old scars. Be careful to stretch a new scar along its length rather than crosswise so that you do not pull the wound open as you stretch. An older scar that is well healed is no longer in danger of ripping open and should be stretched in all directions.

If a scar is not rehabilitated, it will leave a permanent feeling of stiffness, becoming a blockage or interference to the natural flow of the surrounding tissue. This sounds harmless—but it can become very serious. Each scar is different and so has different degrees of seriousness—its location, its size, and the reason behind the surgery all factor into its long-term impact. But all scars must be treated to avoid a lifetime of pain.

When the range of motion of any body part is limited by a scar, the surrounding muscles and other soft tissue will atrophy, the connective tissue that coats each cell hardens, creating new scar tissue. The area of the initial scar becomes even more immobilized and can even be hard to the touch.

The initial discomfort and stiffness from a scar is generally not the cause of the pain. The pain comes because of a muscular imbalance that is caused by the scar. If the scar is not sufficiently rehabilitated, this can be the start of a slippery slope. One scar can set off a chain reaction of scarring and immobility that leads to a lifetime of chronic pain.

Surgery

All kinds of surgeries can potentially lead to seemingly unrelated issues of immobility and chronic pain. In addition to the inevitable scar tissue that results from the surgical incision, surgery often changes the length of tendons and muscles, creating an imbalance in the movement of a joint. These repercussions of scars and imbalances often lead to chronic pain, which needs to be prevented with daily exercise.

Breast cancer surgery, for example, is known to cause adhesive capsulitis (frozen shoulder) and chronic shoulder pain. Pancreatic cancer surgery can lead to chronic chest, shoulder, and upper-body pain.

Spinal fusion surgery—a procedure that typically involves a bone graft or a metal implant in the spine to immobilize damaged vertebrae—may successfully eliminate the initial back pain but often brings with it unforeseen side effects, such as when the fused-together vertebrae rub painfully together. The worst side effect of spinal fusion surgery is the physical immobility of the surrounding and attaching muscles and tendons. This happens because spinal fusion sends a psychological message to the person that says he or she cannot or should not bend his or her spine. After surgery, many patients are afraid of damaging their spine, so they take extreme precautions not to bend or twist it. The fear of bending and twisting leads to weakening, atrophying, and shrinking of the spinal muscles. What such patients forget is that they have thirty-three vertebrae—if three vertebrae have been fused, they still have thirty vertebra to safely bend and twist with! Fusing of two or three vertebra is just a tiny part of the whole. To prevent additional spinal muscle imbalances, it's important to keep moving and not become paralyzed by fear.

Injuries Old and New

Unfortunately, injuries are part of the human experience, the ultimate price of living a full, active life. Accidents happen! Very few people have not suffered at least one injury—especially in childhood or young adulthood, when we are afraid of nothing and prepared to try anything. Some of us who suffered injuries in our youth are still dealing with the pain thirty, forty, and fifty years later. Often this is because when we are younger, we don't think twice about the long-term consequences of a sprain or a torn muscle or a broken bone, and we're too impatient to spend the necessary time to recover and rehabilitate properly.

Honestly, you would not believe the stories I have heard. People have told me all kinds of crazy tales—of taking a bad fall while skiing and then getting up to finish the run; of tearing a ligament and going on to complete the marathon; of twisting an ankle and finishing the competition; of sustaining a concussion and staying in the game. I've even heard of a motorcycle rider who dislocated his shoulder in an accident and then got back on his bike to ride for several thousand more miles!

Life is too much fun, and we shouldn't miss any of it because of pain from injuries. Injuries are common, and the human body is designed to repair most of them—but we don't always give the body a chance to do its natural healing magic. In addition, many doctors don't know how to take the step from healing an injury to rehabilitating the body back to its original state.

The good news is that even old injuries that have been ignored for decades can be rehabilitated. It's always the same story of imbalances leading to damaged joints. And it's always the same solution: to rebalance by carefully stretching and strengthening the full body.

Obesity

Obesity has become a major health epidemic, so I would be remiss not to touch on it in a conversation about the causes of chronic pain. Excessive weight is lethal for joint health. Our joints have the ability to last at least 125 years, well beyond our life expectancy. However, no matter how perfect any piece of engineering may be, joints cannot survive when excessive weight is placed on them. As a result, the obesity epidemic has caused an explosion in the number of hip and knee replacements.

Obviously, obesity is a very difficult condition to reverse. Of those who manage to lose 5 percent of their weight, only one in 20 can maintain that weight loss for longer than 5 years.[4] We can see from the recidivism rate that losing weight is not just a matter of reducing the calorie intake. But the severity of the health impact on an obese person's ability to comfortably and safely move around cannot be overstated. We need to move to keep our vital organs healthy, yet movement can feel awkward, uncomfortable, and, when the joints begin to wear out, painful.

If you are overweight, your joints will eventually become damaged from the unrelenting pressure put on them. Our muscles are designed to be strong, but they are not designed with enough strength to support an obese body. The truth is that carrying around extra pounds is exactly that: carrying. Whether you are carrying luggage, groceries, or your own excessive weight, repetitive carrying will place excessive stress on your muscles and joints and wear them out. There is no way to avoid or deny that obesity is very damaging to the joints.

Obesity also sets in motion a series of chain reactions that serve as a precursor to chronic pain—movement becomes tiring and painful, so the person becomes sedentary; the muscles weaken from a lack of movement; the connective tissue hardens; the immobile muscles atrophy; and atrophied muscles result in fewer mitochondria to burn calories. All of this leads to chronic pain felt throughout the body—everything hurts, all the time.

When my clients lose weight, they are always overjoyed at how much better they feel in their bodies, and how much less pain they experience on a daily basis. Many people don't realize how much joint pain they've been living with until it disappears.

Poor Circulation

Blood is a life force that courses through our veins and arteries, nourishing and cleansing our cells, and feeding our brain. Simply stated, without blood we would die—and without good circulation our cells do slowly die.

Plaque that builds up in the arteries of the limbs can result in peripheral artery disease (PAD), which causes numbness, cell death, spasm, and blood clots. Narrowed or blocked arteries may also cause problems in the intestines or kidneys, and can decrease blood flow to the limbs and outer extremities.

The laws of atrophy and cell death apply to all cells of the human body, including the cells of the veins and arteries. As plaque builds inside the walls of the arteries, the arterial muscles become inhibited from movement. Immobility always leads to cell death, atrophy, and a hardening of the tissue—the arterial wall is no different. This is where gentle, deep, full-body stretching brings an important benefit.

We need good circulation in order to prevent many serious diseases and much pain. Poor circulation limits the body's ability to heal itself. Blood circulates into every cell of the body, which means that we must maintain strong circulation in every part of the body. Large, full-body stretching movements are the most effective way to flush the blood through every artery and vein in the body for the maintenance of a healthy circulatory system.

CHAPTER 4

Using the Essentrics Method to Become Forever Painless

The human body is designed to function like a magnificent orchestra—every instrument is essential to create the beautiful melody of a vibrant life. If one instrument is not properly tuned or plays out of rhythm, the entire symphony is disrupted. When we have muscle atrophy or imbalances, blockages in connective tissue, joint damage, or other causes of chronic pain, the beautiful melodies of life become completely discordant.

Luckily we are the conductors of this orchestra, and we have the power to restore harmony within our bodies. By following the gentle exercises in this book for 20 to 30 minutes a day, we can help the systems of our body play together beautifully. Essentrics was designed to fine-tune every instrument in the human body, allowing our muscles, bones, joints, and tissues to play as they should. The result for us is increased mobility, flexibility, and pain-free living.

Before we get into the details of the program, let's take a closer look at why this type of approach is so effective.

The Goldilocks Balance:
Equal Strength and Flexibility

Soon after *Classical Stretch* went national on the PBS network in 1999, I started receiving emails from fans who told me that their chronic pain had disappeared and they no longer needed to take their pain medication. I was thrilled, of course, but at that point I didn't fully understand this unintended side effect of the program—I didn't yet realize its full potential for healing. In fact, at the time, I was still brainwashed by the prevailing "no pain, no gain" philosophy of the fitness industry, under the delusion that all exercise should cause some amount of pain or discomfort—indeed, that pain was a signal you were doing it *right*, that you were working hard and pushing yourself to full capacity.

How wrong I was!

Now I know that the definition of a healthy body is a just-right balance between strength and flexibility—the Goldilocks balance. To make movement easy and effortless, muscles must be as strong as they are flexible. Pain-free movement, by necessity, involves both healthy joints and healthy muscles. A healthy joint must be able to bend or rotate, just as the glassy head on each adjoining bone slides or glides over a well-lubricated surface. Healthy muscles must be capable of easily, efficiently, and smoothly moving the joints. Any interference with these smoothly moving joints will lead to pain.

How does your current exercise program make you feel? Essentrics instructors pride themselves on the fact that, even after an hour-long class, none of our students are in pain, either during the class or hours later. What they feel instead is stronger, more flexible, and more energetic. This is how you should *always* feel after exercising. If you are in pain, remember that that's a warning sign from the body that something isn't right! Ignoring or "powering through" your pain simply sets you up for more pain down the line.

Essentrics will help you pay attention to the subtle signals your body is sending you, helping you realign your spine, rebalance your muscle groups, and release long-standing blockages in your soft tissue. And, as a bonus, not only will it help relieve your pain, it will also help you achieve the long, lean, and toned look that you might have been trying to develop in more dangerous, less effective ways.

Two Types of Strengthening: Concentric and Eccentric

Every muscle is made up of tens of thousands of fibers, or filaments, that shorten or lengthen each time we move. These fibers are designed to be strong *and* mobile, the true yin-yang of our musculature. Two types of exercise techniques strengthen the muscles: concentric and eccentric. Concentric training, the most common type, shortens these fibers as they are being strengthened. Eccentric training, the kind featured in Essentrics, lengthens the fibers while strengthening them.

Both concentric and eccentric movements are part of our everyday lives. Getting out of bed requires us to bend our knees and lean forward (concentric) as we stand upright (eccentric). We do concentric movements when we lift heavy loads: groceries, books, briefcases, heavy purses, and so on.

If we're not careful about getting an equal amount of eccentric movement to offset the concentric movement, we can end up with two very different and very serious problems: semi-immobilized connective tissue and compressed joints.

In addition to the functional concentric movements in our daily lives, there's also the more concentrated concentric movements we engage in when we exercise. In sports and fitness, most joint damage is the result of exercise programs that focus on concentric movements. Weight lifting, running, racket sports, and high-impact or interval training all use concentric movement. Every time you lift a weight, do a push-up or chin-up, or hold a static pose in yoga, you are shortening your muscles.

When a fitness program isn't balanced with eccentric training, the muscles will shorten and become less and less flexible. The shortening of muscles around joints squeezes the joints tightly together, leading to joint damage and pain. Overstrengthened, shortened muscles have little to zero flexibility, making them (and the attached tendons) prone to injury. This is the primary reason why millions of athletes, from casual to professional, suffer from knee, hip, and foot pain, and have shin splints and torn meniscuses, ACLs, and groin muscles.

Inside our muscle cells, thousands of muscle fibers are constantly stretching and recoiling. Repeated concentric training compresses the muscle fibers in their shortened position, limiting their ability to stretch. When our cells cannot effortlessly glide in and out of their protective sheaths, the connective tissue surrounding them begins to congeal. As I noted in chapter 2, this hardening of the connective tissue leads to muscle immobility, cell death, and pain—not good at all.

In contrast to concentric training, eccentric training maintains the full range of motion of all muscles. Also, no joint damage can occur where the muscles are strong within their length, comfortably preventing joint compression. Healthy muscles have flexibility built into their strength so that their smoothly sliding movements can continue into our golden years. The combination of these optimal conditions is called eccentric strength, in which the power is imbedded within the flexibility.

The goal is to build muscles that have the same type of strength that you see in a flexible tree branch. Consider this: A five-foot tree branch can withstand much more pressure than a five-foot piece of wood of the same diameter. If you could fix a five-foot tree branch between two points and smash down on the branch with a baseball bat—what do you think would happen? Chances are, the branch would bend but not break. But if you were to fix a five-foot piece of solid, inflexible wood between two points and with equal force smash it with a baseball bat, what do you think would happen? I'll tell you—it would definitely break.

Flexibility is part of the strength of the branch, protecting it from nature's forces. Depending on the type of training you do, your muscles will react similarly to the branch or the long stick. With concentric training, they tear from rigidity. With eccentric training, they yield to force and rebound intact.

How Essentrics Heals the Whole Body

Remember: When we stretch, we are stretching not only muscle but also connective tissue. Fascia, the component of the connective tissue system that comprises much of the human body, forms a continuous tensional network, covering and connecting every organ, muscle, and muscle fiber. This network imparts a continuous tension to the system—any pressure applied to the body is distributed equally throughout the system, which allows us to withstand tremendous force instead of absorbing it in one local area.

Rather than being composed of simple sheets of biological tissue draped over our bones and muscles and stuffed between our organs, fascia is flexible and rich in collagen, the substance that gives our youthful skin its glow. Fascia is like a fabulously dynamic and responsive bodysuit! Long-term and regular practice of eccentric stretching has a positive impact on the architecture of the fascia, helping maintain its youthful elasticity and improving the connections and the communication among all of our bodily systems.

Slow, dynamic stretching is especially effective in the hydration and renewal of fascia, which is made up of free-moving and bound water molecules. The human body is awash in fluids—water comprises about 60 percent of our total body mass. Just as the squeezing of a damp sponge moves the moisture from one place to another, the strain of stretching pushes fascial liquid from areas where it may have congealed out into the network, dispersing the fluids, keeping the connective tissue moist and pliable, and refreshing other neglected areas that don't have adequate hydration. The dynamic stretching found in Essentrics reaches into parts of the body not targeted by everyday movement or by most other exercise programs.

Essentrics focuses on large, full-body movements—the kind of movements that work on all planes, somewhat similar to tai chi sequences. The scientific term for these movements is *isotonic*. In contrast to static *isometric* exercises, in which the angle of the joints and the length of the muscles do not change during the contraction, isotonic movements mimic everyday life and are widely accepted as the safest and most effective way to train the human body. They are so easy to do that literally anyone at any age and any level of fitness can do them. They have been scientifically designed to stretch and strengthen, stimulating a biochemical reaction that combats cell death and atrophy in every muscle and joint chain in the body.

Large weight-free full-body movements are the most effective method to stretch and strengthen the entire musculature while stimulating connective tissue that covers, envelopes, and surrounds our cells. The movements in Essentrics engage all 650 muscles, from fingers to toes and everything in between. No one muscle group is developed more than the others. All muscles are trained to do equal work so that no imbalance injuries can occur.

For most of human history, up until quite recently, we have engaged in these types of movements without giving them a second thought. Our mothers and grandmothers certainly got plenty of eccentric exercise—activities like gardening, hanging laundry on a clothesline, or washing windows and floors. These simple daily chores were full-body eccentric movements. But our lifestyles have changed to the point where many of these activities have become obsolete, completed by machines, or are outsourced to others—so we no longer have the daily opportunity to simultaneously stretch and strengthen our muscles. Because we are no longer required to move to the extent we once were, it is therefore vital for us to consciously create opportunities for full-body movement. If we don't, we risk overusing some parts of our bodies while barely using other parts. Over time, these imbalances translate into hip, shoulder, back, and foot pain.

Every cell in our body directly or indirectly affects every other cell. The brain talks to every cell, and the blood circulates to every cell. The digestive system nourishes every cell, and the endocrine system regulates every cell. Our body is a single human unit.

This is one of the major reasons why large, full-body movements are so beneficial for our health and well-being. When you do a full-body movement, such as picking up a box from the floor and putting it in a high cupboard, almost every cell in your body has been stimulated. These full-body movements keep the inter- and intracellular communication channels activated, open, and clear.

I meet people who walk a lot, some even one to two hours a day. Walking is great exercise for the hips and maybe the cardiovascular system if the walking is fast enough and uphill—but it engages only about 50 percent of the body's actual musculature. I have no-

WHY NOT WEIGHTS?

In a gym setting, a trainer might recommend that you lift a three-, four-, or five-pound barbell to strengthen your muscles. Or in a yoga or Pilates class, you might be asked to hold poses until your form breaks. Weight training and holding are concentric exercises.

Most adults weigh between 130 and 200 pounds just standing on the ground. That's already a lot of weight to be lifting and lowering, bending and twisting. What on earth will an extra 3 to 10 pounds do to strengthen the muscles? The answer is very little extra strengthening—however, after enough repetitions, your joints will become compressed and painful.

We forget that we *are* a weight—every part of our body weighs something. Even our baby finger weighs something! So unless you are planning to become a professional athlete, you don't need to lift weights. You could spend hours doing isolated weight training and stretching and still not achieve the same well-balanced strength and flexibility that 20 minutes of full-body movements can provide. We can tone our muscles and become extremely strong just by doing large, full-body movements.

ticed that people who use walking as their exclusive exercise often have large tummies, weak core muscles, and underdeveloped arm muscles. That's because their upper body doesn't get any exercise from walking.

When I gently suggest this, some people blame their heavy bellies and weak upper bodies on the aging process. They're convinced that their hours of walking are all the exercise they need to stay fit. But the human body doesn't lie. If you don't use some parts of your body, those unused parts will weaken and atrophy. Strong muscles give us our shape, and when our muscles weaken, our body shape changes. Aging is not the cause of weakness—disuse is. Remember: Use it or lose it. The only way to keep your entire body strong, fit, and pain-free is to engage every part of it on a regular basis.

Gentle Movement Heals Pain

You actually build strength much more quickly when you are *not* in pain than when you are—especially if you are recovering from an injury. But that doesn't mean you should wait until you are pain-free to begin exercising. When you have an injury or are suffering from chronic pain, regular gentle exercise is *essential* to prevent atrophy while rebuilding healthy tissue.

Gentle exercise helps create new patterns in the brain, erasing the previous pain loop that we know is a key component of chronic pain. As we've discussed, chronic pain can be the function of a faulty pain-signaling system: the brain can continue to receive pain messages long after the major damage has been healed. This is not a psychological phenomenon—the pain signal is actually real, kept alive by the self-perpetuating biochemical loop, like a broken record that continues to skip. This type of pain is common among people who have ignored injuries throughout their lives. After they have ignored the messages for years, their brain becomes programmed to play *only* the pain message. The nervous system begins to act like an ignored child who throws a tantrum in order to get her parent's attention!

Essentrics weaves many different methods of flexibility training into every workout to interrupt this loop and achieve pain relief. However, when we are trying to break the neurological pain loop, it is essential to practice all of the following techniques in a gentle, relaxed manner:

1. RELAXATION INTO DEEP ECCENTRIC FLEXIBILITY. Relaxing to release the tension while slowly moving is one of the most powerful ways to gently, safely, and rapidly increase flexibility and strength while reprogramming the pain loop. It is part of the eccentric school of exercises, as it strengthens while increasing flexibility.

2. BREATHING. Deep breathing is a powerful, natural way to help release tension in locked muscle fibers and fasciae. Deep breathing helps release tension and thus permits other forms of flexibility to take over, such as eccentric or passive stretching.

3. REBALANCING THE MUSCLES. You are only as loose as your tightest muscle. Your body is one large, interdependent unit of 650 muscles. Any unbalanced muscle will lead to other imbalances in seemingly unrelated parts of your body, and those imbalances, in turn, lead to potential damage, pain, and injury.

4. ECCENTRIC TRAINING: Lengthening the muscle fibers simultaneously increases both flexibility and strength, which decompresses joints.

5. PASSIVE FLEXIBILITY. When no strength is required, we can simply let our muscles slowly release their tension into deeper flexibility—such as in floor work, when we are lying on our back and pulling our leg toward our chest either with our hands or with the aid of a stretch band. The legs should be as relaxed as those of a rag doll as they are being passively stretched.

6. PNF FLEXIBILITY. Proprioceptive neuromuscular facilitation (PNF) is a technique that works on the neurological system to trick the muscles into releasing tension. Most people unconsciously hold tension in their muscles, which makes the muscles difficult to stretch. Physical therapists often use PNF when helping clients recover from injury or surgery. It releases contracted muscles, enabling stiff muscles to be stretched. PNF is a four-step procedure of (1) contract the muscle, (2) release the contraction, (3) relax the muscle more, and (4) stretch the muscle. It is safe, achieves rapid results, and feels really good.

7. MOVING WITHIN A STRETCH. This method rebalances and engages all the muscles around a joint, as it helps all muscles to become equally stretched.

All these flexibility methods are helpful, and each is done for a specific purpose. When combined correctly, they work together synergistically, like the ingredients of a gourmet recipe, offering you perfect results.

Don't Be Afraid to Move

In order to achieve lasting pain relief, you must unlock the healing potential within your cells through movement. Unfortunately, many chronic pain sufferers fear that moving will make their pain worse. It's a legitimate concern, because it's true—most of the time when they move, they do feel pain. This creates a natural dilemma: they've been told by their doctors to be more active, yet even a modest amount of activity causes pain. They don't want to trigger the pain, so they don't do the one thing that will get rid of the pain. I found myself in this dilemma after my own surgeries—so it's no surprise to me that most people don't know how to exercise when they are in pain.

The way out of this dilemma is to move slowly and to stop every time the pain starts. This disrupts the pain loop from the muscle to the brain. When you move yet stop just before you trigger the pain message, your brain will no longer connect that movement to pain. Note: This works only if the cause of pain has been totally healed but the pain *message* has not gone away. There will also probably be some areas where the pain persists—those are areas that still need to be healed.

Exercising in a pain-free state is possible as long as you are prepared to work like a rag doll, feeling as though you are being lazy. I call the fully relaxed, rag-doll state the "healing state." The rag-doll state is the most powerful healing state you can use, as it is working in harmony with the neurological system. The rag-doll state stops all the natural protective reflexes from contracting the muscles; in doing so, it permits a flow of healing fluids into the pain-stricken region. Gentle, pain-free movement is healing movement. It heals the injuries and resets the broken pain loop.

If you are suffering from chronic pain, the only road to a pain-free body is correct, gentle, full-body rebalancing exercises. There is no pill you can take, no surgery you can undergo, and no amount of massages, hot baths, or passive treatments that will get rid of imbalanced muscles and poor alignment. Correct exercise is the only way to heal your body.

You have two choices: to remain in pain or to get out of pain. Getting out of pain requires a commitment to 30 minutes of daily exercise.

HOW TO BREAK THE PAIN LOOP

I have found this simple trick to be quite successful in helping many people break the pain loop: Stand with your legs in a comfortable stance, not too wide but not too close together. Hold your arms at your side, breathing easily while relaxing all your muscles. Wait until you are completely relaxed and pain-free before starting to move. Then start to slowly and gently sway your body from side to side. If you are still pain-free, add a slight rotation in both directions, twisting around the spine. The moment you feel even the slightest twinge of pain, stop and return to the beginning position, where you were pain-free. The trick in changing a neurological pain loop is not to permit your body to experience pain.

Some people experience pain the moment they move—but there is usually a place, as you begin to move, where you are pain-free. If that's your case, move a tiny bit and stop before the pain triggers. Hold and relax in the pain-free point for a few seconds; this is generally long enough for the message that you are still pain-free at this spot to reach your brain. Then, start moving again. These incremental steps of stop and start within a pain-free zone take time. But once you have shown the brain that movement doesn't automatically equate with danger, you will soon be able to move without pain.

We want the pain message to be triggered only when there is danger—and not trigger because of an endless loop. It takes patience to lay down a new pathway for the brain to follow. To reverse pain loops in all your daily activities, you might have to go through the motions of standing, sitting, walking, and getting out of a car slowly, retraining the brain to see that you are safe when you do them.

You may need to repeat this process a few times, but the amazing thing is that when you take the time to show your body that it's not in danger when you move, the pain loop turns off rapidly.

NOTE: This trick works only if the original damage is actually healed but the pain message is stuck in a loop. If your body still has some real damage, the pain you feel will be *real* and this trick won't work.

You're Ready to Begin

hope by now I've convinced you that correct, gentle movement is the best and fastest way to heal your chronic pain. Even if you remain skeptical, ask yourself: *What do I really have to lose?* Let's get started with your workouts.

Before each sequence, it is essential to start with the basic warm-up presented in chapter 5. It will wake up your muscles and joints and get them ready to move comfortably. Once you've completed the brief warm-up, you can select from any of the nine workouts to address the area of your body that has been giving you the most pain. I give you my solemn promise: If you have been struggling with chronic pain of any kind, once you incorporate Essentrics into your daily life and stick with it for a few weeks, your pain will be either greatly diminished or completely gone.

Really!

Believe in yourself and see what your body can do!

Part Two

The Forever Painless Program

CHAPTER 5

The Basic Warm-Up

Twenty years ago, I would never have believed it was possible to achieve profound results with only 30 minutes of gentle exercise a day—it went against everything I had been taught about how much time and effort was required to achieve real changes. That was before I understood the science of the human body, and before I understood how to combine anatomy, neurology, and physiology with correct movement. It was also before *Classical Stretch* had aired on PBS for seventeen years and I had received thousands of emails from people whose lives had been changed simply by doing these workouts.

Since then, I've seen many different types of chronic pain be healed by this program. Even when people have the best surgery and medication, I've found that exercise is essential to finish the job in bringing about total pain relief. Correct movement plays a vital role in the healing process, and the converse is also absolutely true: when exercise is absent, full recovery and long-term pain relief are rarely achieved.

Chapters 6 through 13 each start with stories about people who've used Essentrics to heal their chronic and sometimes debilitating pain. I love these stories; they show the power of courage and commitment, and the determination of the human spirit to overcome seemingly insurmountable obstacles. They encourage and reassure us that, yes, there is always hope. And after years of working with people in pain, I've been surprised and delighted to discover that even when clients are limited in their ability to do the exercises exactly as intended, they're still able to reap the benefits of this program. Perfect form is less important than the action of movement itself. Every part of the human body just needs to move, it's as simple as that!

If you are presently suffering from chronic pain, doing the exercises in this book should reduce or completely rid you of pain. But I urge you to always listen to your body. Remember that you are unique—feel free to tweak the exercises to suit your individual needs. Do only what feels comfortable at this moment in your life. Tomorrow you might feel differently; you can continue to adjust the workouts every day.

To start, find a comfortable, flat space with either a low carpet (not pile) or a bare floor. Remove your shoes and socks. (With bare feet you'll develop greater stability and use more of your full-body muscles.) These workouts can be done in a very small space—just make sure that as you stretch side to side you won't hit anything.

Remember: Don't miss a day! Your body needs these movements every day to start to heal. Do these workouts for about 30 minutes a day, and I promise that you *will* feel a change. Many people feel so good doing them, they'll do the exercises both in the morning and at night. This is completely safe—the program is that gentle!

HOW CAN I STRETCH WHILE I'M IN PAIN?

This is one of our most frequently asked questions. If you're currently in pain, you might wonder, "How can I stretch when it hurts to move?" The answer is: Slowly and gently. You should move in the stretch only up to the point at which you feel pain. At that point, stop until the pain subsides, then continue. If you are just beginning, you might want to break up the workouts into three or four smaller sessions and do this process for 5 to 10 minutes three or four times a day. Before you know it, the initial pain will be gone and you should be able to do the full stretching motion.

The trick is never to push through the pain—*always* stop the moment you feel pain, wait a few seconds for the pain to subside, and then continue. Always move gently. Rough movements will feel like you are ripping something—which you might actually be doing! Slow movements loosen and melt the glued-together connective tissue without tearing it.

When you push your body through pain, instead of stopping at the point of pain, you will actually create *more* future pain by damaging the connective tissue. Remember: Tearing creates scar tissue that in turn restricts the flow of information and nutrients through connective tissue—all of which leads to more physical restriction and pain.

Patience and gentle daily movements are the fastest and safest way to heal. Haste makes waste.

Warm-Up Guidelines for All Workouts

The warm-up exercises that follow are designed to increase the circulation of blood and connective tissue fluids in your body while increasing your body's temperature. They gently prepare your muscles for specific movements by releasing tension and improving mobility. They trigger the mitochondria to burn calories, which is what warms the muscles and liberates the joints. Warm-ups loosen tight fasciae, facilitating the layers of connective tissue to glide effortlessly over the natural surfaces of our muscles, tendons, ligaments, and nerves.

Never skip the warm-up exercises, as they are an essential part of every workout. Your body requires this preparatory phase in order to be fully capable of safely completing the routines.

A few more things to keep in mind as you start your workouts:

NO PAIN, EVER. If at any point a knifelike pain sensation kicks in, immediately stop and return to where you were prior to feeling the pain. Never push through a sharp pain. Always stop and go back to the point where you were just before the pain sensation kicked in. Give your muscles a few seconds to let the pain signal subside before moving again. I can't repeat this critical aspect of healing enough: *Always exercise in a pain-free zone.* Only after you have become pain-free should you change your mode of exercising from protection to full energy. Listen to your body. It will tell you when you are ready to work harder and with more intensity. And when your chronic pain has gone, you can and should work to your full safe capacity. When you are pain-free, you can go back to doing any sport and activity you love, as long as you continue to do regular rebalancing exercises.

STAY RELAXED. Warm-up movements should be performed in as relaxed a mode as possible. Be careful not to hold your joints stiffly. To avoid stiffness, release any grip that the muscles might have on the joints that will prevent the joints from moving loosely. Focus on relaxing, bending, twisting, and moving every joint possible. One good trick in helping relax the full body is to focus on relaxing your fingers. If your fingers are relaxed, it is difficult to tighten your shoulders and upper-back muscles. Look at yourself in a mirror to check that you are actually twisting, bending, and rotating your spine, and you're not moving it as one rigid rod. (Mirrors can be excellent teaching tools!) Most people have a great deal of trouble relaxing; it can be more challenging than strengthening is. But only when you can easily relax your muscles will you be able to completely strengthen them. So spend as much time as you need focused on relaxing.

KEEP THE ENTIRE SOLES OF YOUR FEET ON THE GROUND. Most people walk with their ankles rolling toward the inside or outside of their feet. Before you begin your exercises every day, look at your feet and make sure that the full soles are flat on the ground. Being aware that correct alignment of the bones of your feet will help you slowly rebalance your full body. You will find that standing flat on your feet is not as easy, and will not feel as natural, as it sounds—some muscles will pull you to one side, making it challenging to get the feet flat. Take your time; it may take several weeks before you rebalance the muscles of your feet to the point where standing flat is comfortable. As you place your foot on the ground during the side-to-side steps, check that you actually put the full sole of your foot flat on the ground. Standing correctly on your feet will change how your knees, hips, and spine feel. It will also help you gain more energy and control your weight more easily. The benefits of standing flat on the soles of your feet will ripple throughout your entire skeleton, relieving pain all the way up your spine through to your hands and fingers.

USE THE CHAIR SPARINGLY. While you'll notice that many of the exercises feature the use of a chair for stability, the less you rely upon the chair, the more likely your balance reflexes (the nerves that trigger muscle reactions and balance reflexes) will strengthen. If your reflexes are not stimulated regularly, they will shrivel and atrophy. "Use it or lose it" applies to our nerve cells as much as to all other cells in the body! The best way to regain poor balance is to stimulate the balance reflexes. Just let yourself wobble a bit and even lose your balance slightly, as the wobbling sends valuable balance messages to the brain.

KEEP YOUR STANCE WIDE. In side-to-side steps, also check the width of your stance. Try to avoid short sideways strides, unless a wider stride is painful—but that's not likely to be the case for most of us. With every passing decade, we tend to use our body a little bit less, and that includes shortening our strides, whether side to side or front to back while walking. Remember: Your muscles will shrink if you don't use them. Consciously work on getting back that youthful stride!

USEFUL EQUIPMENT

For all of the Essentrics exercises, you may want to gather the following to have on hand close by:

- A CHAIR. If you are unstable on your feet, need a cane while walking, or generally have a fear of losing your balance, please have a chair nearby. Use it only when it is specified in the exercise description, or when absolutely necessary. Relying upon a chair when you don't really need one will lessen the effectiveness of the exercises.

- A THICK (½-INCH), FIRM MAT. Avoid a mat that is too thin, too soft, or too squishy. You may not need this in a carpeted room. Use only if you are uncomfortable standing on the bare floor.

- A RISER. Useful for elevating your sitting height during some floor exercises, light-weight, wide, firm foam risers are available at fitness supply stores or websites. However, several thick encyclopedias could also serve as excellent risers as they are wide and solid. The height of risers changes according to each student's needs. Some people need to elevate their sitting position by only 2 inches while others need as much as one foot.

- A HEMORRHOID CUSHION. This round, ring-shaped cushion has a hole in the middle. Do not purchase the inflatable ones. The correct ones are made of a firm foam.

- A FIRM STRETCH BAND. Stretch bands—also called exercise bands, sports bands, or resistance bands—come in different levels of resistance.

BEND YOUR KNEES. Always bend your knees when shifting your weight in Essentrics, from lunges, warm-ups, steps, or any other weight shifts. Never step on straight legs. Not only is landing on straight legs hard on the joints, it also puts unnecessary stress on your spine. I promise that your knees won't break if you bend them carefully.

Bend your knees as deeply as possible when doing all the exercises that require bending your knees. Without even thinking about it, most of us try not to bend our knees, because bending them is more tiring than keeping them straight! The deeper we bend the knees, the harder we are working—but human beings instinctively look for the easiest way to move. Both athletes and seniors are equally guilty of this, so be vigilant with your-self and bend those knees. Find the degree of knee bend that doesn't hurt, and use that as your normal level. This counts even if you have chronic knee pain—you will never get rid of knee pain if you don't bend your knees when exercising! The less you bend the knees, the faster the muscles around them will atrophy, causing even more pain. The bonus for bending your knees is that you will burn more calories and gain more muscle tone!

Don't forget to breathe—and keep breathing. Before starting to exercise, take a few slow, deep breaths. Count to 6 slowly as you inhale and exhale. This simple exercise will calm both your muscles and your mind, preparing them to work in a relaxed state. While doing your warm-up exercises, continue to be aware of your breathing. As you focus on moving, make sure you aren't holding your breath. Lots of people unconsciously hold their breath while exercising! Breathing deeply will drive oxygen into your bloodstream so that it can be absorbed into the muscle cells, giving them and you additional fuel. Within seconds, you'll feel the energizing effects of the extra oxygen. Your brain will light up and your energy will increase!

A Word about "Repeated" Exercises

By now you know that correct exercise is not only about the exercises themselves, but much more about how you actually *do* the movements. In order to maximize your benefits safely, you need to know exactly when to relax, stretch, contract, or release tension, and so on. This complex approach is one reason why the Essentrics program is so effective in relieving pain and rebalancing the full body. The human body is complex!

In the chapters that follow, you will notice certain exercises that may *seem* similar to exercises in other chapters. However, the specific instructions for each will vary based on the focus and intent of that sequence. For example, in a hip sequence, you may be instructed to contract, relax, align, inhale, move slowly, wiggle and twist, and pull different parts of your body—all at the same time. Exercises with the same gross motor movements may appear in other sequences, but the specific technique instructions may be slightly different.

The best comparison to be made for understanding the value of using a multitude of techniques is of cooking with exercising. When working with identical ingredients, a chef has a wide variety of technical choices. A potato, for example, may be boiled, baked, roasted, fried, or sautéed. The techniques used in cooking the potato give different results. With Essentrics, the benefits in each sequence rest not in the overall movements but in the technical instructions that fine-tune the sequences to each condition or body region.

The second reason that we often use the same exercises for seemingly separate body parts is that Essentrics is a full-body program. We know that every muscle in our body is either directly or indirectly related to every other muscle. If the muscles of your calf are tight, then the stiffness will spiral from your calf up your leg and tug on your spine, shoulders, and arms. If your knees are in pain, then you must exercise the chains of your muscles up and down your leg, which include your ankles, knees, hips, and spine. We work the full body to include all muscle chains, because only when the full chains are balanced will the pain be permanently relieved.

Remember, these exercises will wake up your muscles and get your body ready for the more focused workouts. Please do this *every* time and don't skip your warm-up if you are short of time—do only the warm-up if that's all you have time for. This warm-up sequence is an essential component of every workout in chapters 6 to 14.

SIDE-TO-SIDE STEPS

These side-to-side steps will loosen the ankle, leg, and hip muscles while improving your circulation.

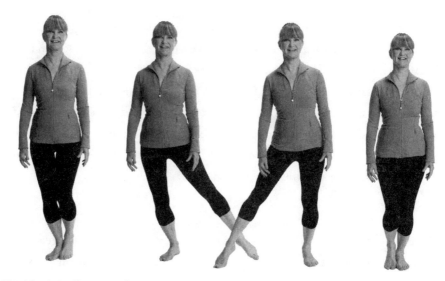

1. Start by bending your knees.

2. Extend your left leg out to the side as far as possible.

3. Step carefully and lightly on your extended foot, trying to pull the weight of your body upward, away from the floor. This pulling-up will stop you from landing with a heavy impact, which is hard on the joints.

4. Bring your feet together and bend your knees, checking that both heels are flat on the ground. Make sure the full weight of your body is evenly distributed over your feet so that your soles are not rolling inward or outward. Rolling will cause joint pain and damage.

5. Alternate from left to right, 16 to 32 times.

HALF-HEIGHT ARM SWINGS WITH SIDE BODY BENDS

These arm swings will improve your circulation while warming up your elbows, spine, torso, hips, and shoulders.

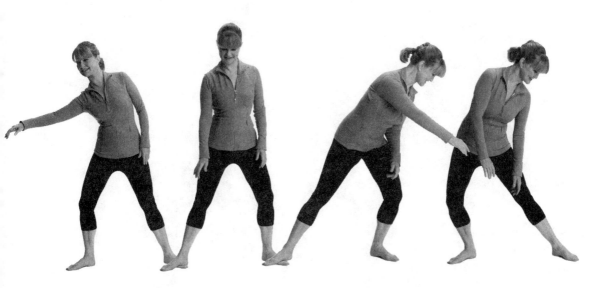

1. Start with feet shoulder-width apart. Shift your weight back and forth, from one foot to the other.

2. Letting your right arm hang loosely from your shoulder, swing it downward in a semicircle as you step from left to right.

3. Your arm should swing in the direction of your body. Bend in a half circle from one side of your body to the other.

4. With every side bend, try to feel your rib muscles stretching. Be aware not to lock your rib cage and move like a rigid box!

5. Ensure that your shoulders and elbows are relaxed throughout the warm-up.

6. Complete 16 swings on each arm while shifting your weight from side to side.

FULL-ARM CIRCLES FROM CEILING TO FLOOR

These full-arm circles are designed to stretch and strengthen your full torso. You will be moving the torso on all planes, from wall to wall and from ceiling to floor.

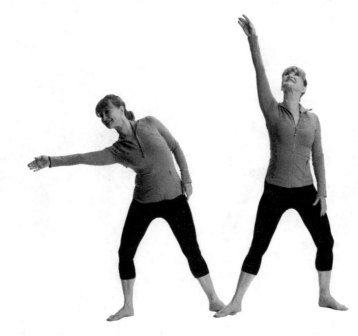

1. Start with your legs in a comfortably wide stance, knees slightly bent.

2. Reach one arm up and imagine that you are drawing a large circle with your arm and torso, following a full circumference from ceiling to floor.

3. Stay relaxed throughout the movements—particularly relax your shoulders and elbows.

4. Focus on breathing deeply throughout the swings.

5. Don't rush. Take your time to move carefully and fully control every movement.

6. Keep the movement controlled; never fling your body or use momentum as you do the circles.

7. Complete 4 large circles with each arm.

THROWING A FRISBEE

The spine is designed to rotate in many directions. This exercise will warm up and loosen the many muscles of your spine, allowing it to rotate comfortably in any direction.

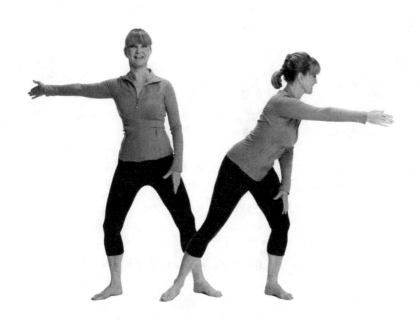

1. Begin by standing in a comfortably wide stance. Extend one arm sideways and bend your knees.

2. Reach across your body, toward the other side of the room.

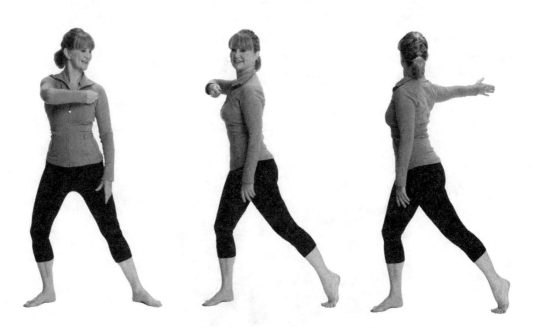

3. Imagine that you are throwing a Frisbee.

4. Throw the imaginary Frisbee behind you, toward the back of the room.

5. As you throw, turn your head to look behind you, in the direction of where you are throwing the imaginary Frisbee.

6. Lift your back heel as you rotate your body (which will release any excessive tension on the spine).

7. Repeat this 4 times on each side.

8. Complete the entire sequence twice, for a total of 8 times on each side.

RAISING AND LOWERING THE ARMS WHILE BENDING SLIGHTLY FORWARD

This final warm-up is designed to relax all of the muscles that help your spine bend forward. We have the tendency to tense or grip our bodies throughout our day, making us uncomfortable and prone to back spasms. This exercise will help you release spinal tension.

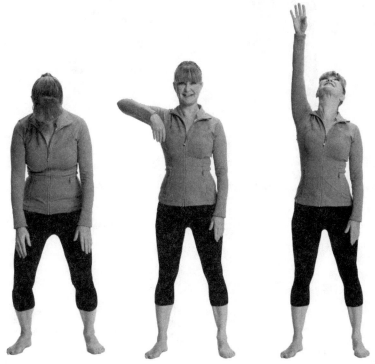

1. Before beginning, breathe deeply 4 times, and focus on relaxing your muscles.
2. Stand with feet shoulder-width apart, bending slightly forward, rounding the back with your knees bent.
3. Allow your arms to hang loosely at your sides.
4. With the fingertips of one hand, trace the length of your body, all the way up.

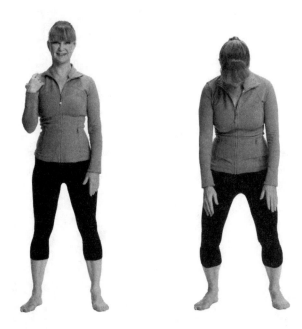

5. Finish with that hand reaching toward the ceiling.

6. Slowly lower your arm, bending your elbow and relaxing your shoulder muscles as your arm comes down.

7. Return to your starting position, and begin again with the opposite arm.

8. Repeat 16 times, alternating arms each time.

CHAPTER 6

The Foot and Ankle Workout

n 1999, the Canadian athlete Jonathon Power became the first North American to be ranked the world's number one squash player, an accomplishment he achieved several more times throughout his career. But even for the most focused, dedicated, and gifted athlete, being at the top of a competitive sport is a constant mental and physical challenge. When I first met Jonathon in 2000, he had a troubling array of physical problems. He had even considered leaving the pro circuit.

Jonathon was a child when he started playing squash and was soon putting in hours of daily practice and winning national junior titles. He dropped out of high school to work on his game, turning pro at age sixteen.

A fast, aerobically intense, physically grueling game of infinite combinations and angles, squash is demanding on the joints, which are subject to relentless compression and pounding; it is particularly punishing on the knees, lower vertebrae, and hips. Injuries are common among squash players, and pain is a constant companion, on court and off, for top competitive players.

When I met Jonathon his goal wasn't to eliminate the pain; he'd lived with pain all his life. Instead, he wanted to eliminate the problem that was shutting down his body. His mind could tolerate the pain, but his body, refusing to accept any more abuse, had forced him to stop with full-blown back and groin spasms. "By the time I got to the round that I really needed to win, my body was so beat up I couldn't continue," he said.

Before working with me, Jonathon had worked with a chiropractor, an acupuncturist, and a soft-tissue therapist. And, of course, he had regular message therapy and was proficient at standard athletic stretches as well as the art of icing. But when Jonathon moved back to his native Montreal from Toronto, he left that team of healers behind him. Once he started working with me, he felt no need to have such a team on hand. "The only time I ever saw those guys after that was if I was out with a tear or with injuries that needed to be dealt with by physiotherapy," he said.

Jonathon explained that his trouble originated in his hips: "The hips are where all your speed is. And when they got bound up, that gave me back spasms and a whole bunch of other problems." However, I got to the root of Jonathon's back spasms by working on his feet first, before starting on his hips and the rest of his body.

Most people, including athletes, are unaware of the major role that their feet (including their toes) and ankles play in their overall full-body mobility. In my experience working with high-performance athletes, I have found that little to no training is done to keep their feet mobile and strong. Most athletes wear running shoes, boots, or skates all day, every day, never taking them off to train the hundreds of muscles of their feet. This results in "locked," prematurely atrophied ankles and feet. Many high-performance athletes, and weekend warriors, too, end up with weak feet, calves, and shins. This leads to shin splints, inflammation of the groin and hip muscles, and back spasms. I can almost always trace the source of shoulder, back, and hip pain to immobilized feet and ankles. Many times, when we fix the feet, the other problems go away.

If your toes are immobile, you are almost guaranteed to suffer from a chain reaction of contracted muscles from your feet to your fingers. Where the chain reaction lodges and creates inflammation depends on the individual, but back spasms and hip pain are often directly related to immobile ankles and feet. This was Jonathon's case.

When I began working with him, the first thing I noticed was that his toes and ankles were almost 100 percent immobile. On a day-to-day basis, he lived with a level of pain that would have incapacitated most people. Once he understood that he could conquer this pain with correct exercise, his devotion to reversing it showed me that his status as the longest-reigning world squash champion in history was no coincidence. He put in the time necessary to fix his body, and that was a lot!

During our first few days of training, we spent hours working almost exclusively on regaining the full strength and mobility of his bare feet, using many of the exercises offered in this chapter. As the muscles in his feet relaxed and lengthened, so did the chains of muscles throughout his body.

For six weeks, we continued working daily on deep, full-body Essentrics stretches with an emphasis on hips and feet. Jonathon generally did 90 minutes a day with me, after a full day of his regular squash training. "The reason I did it was because I was seeing results so soon; I would say after a week or two into it," he said. "And then I was hooked because of the freedom in my body—I was finally able to move the way I used to."

I traveled with Jonathon to some key squash matches. His hips regularly got jammed up and locked during the preliminary rounds, so I used Essentrics movement to eliminate his locked hips. "I had other people doing my strength fitness and conditioning, but I had Miranda really keeping my body loose and strong and my reactions fast," he said.

No matter where he was in the world, Jonathon found himself naturally incorporating the Essentrics training into his daily routine. At that point in his life, thanks to Essentrics, Jonathon said, "I was so in tune with my body by then that whenever I felt I needed it, I would just do it."

In 2006, at the age of thirty-one, Jonathan announced his retirement from professional sports. It was one day after he had regained the number one world ranking—to this day, he holds the record as the oldest squash player ever to attain that title.

Pain in your feet and ankles can create problems throughout your body. These exercises can help your foundation, your feet, become strong, flexible, and pain-free.

TOE, ARCH, AND ANKLE STRETCHES

This exercise is designed to relieve foot and ankle pain, such as plantar fasciitis, by helping each individual joint in the foot move effortlessly and with strength and power.

> **EQUIPMENT NOTE:**
>
> **The workout throughout chapter 6 requires a chair. You will need a solid chair with a high back that will not topple over when you put your leg on the seat of the chair, and will be of a comfortable height so that you can hold on to it securely.**

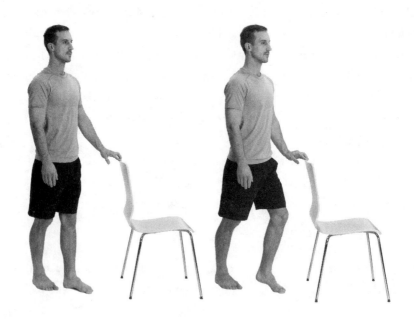

1. Hold the back of your chair with one or both hands.

2. Slowly raise one heel. Be very careful to maintain clean bone alignment—your toes, ankle, and knee should be stacked one above the other, so that the weight of your body can flow effortlessly through the bones of your leg into your foot.

3. Finish the movement by pointing your toes to lift the foot off the ground. Your toes and the arch of your foot should be pointed as much as possible, to stretch the shin.

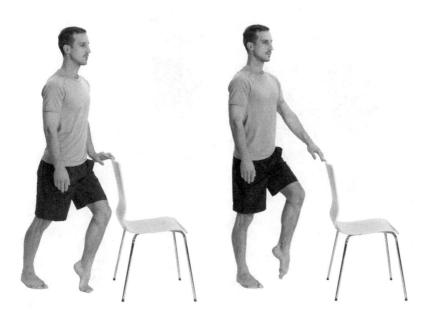

You should feel the muscles across the front of your foot and into your shin being stretched.

4. Reverse the exercise, placing your foot on the ground again, starting the movement with your toes, then your ankle, and finally your heel.

5. Repeat 8 times on each foot.

ANKLE AND FOOT FREESTANDING FLEXION SEQUENCE

This exercise is also designed to relieve foot and ankle pain. Similar to the previous exercise, it's effective in relieving plantar fasciitis.

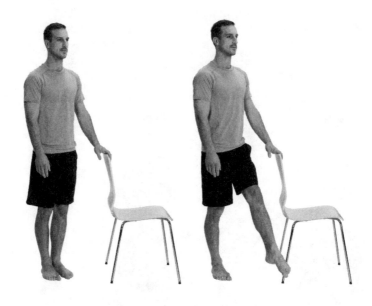

1. Hold the back of your chair with one or both hands.

2. Extending one leg forward, stand straight and point your toes and foot.

3. Note: Be aware not to lean forward or backward, or to sink into your lower spine.

4. Isolate your toes as you flex them; you will feel the muscles of your toes and shin working.

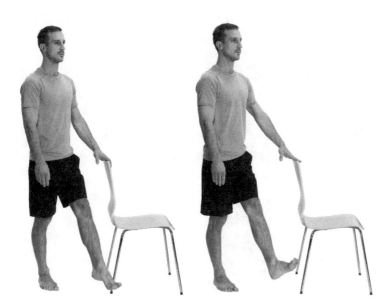

5. Continue flexing the entire ankle; you will feel your calf stretching and your shin contracting.

6. Reverse the movement, starting with your ankle and finishing with your toes.

7. Repeat 4 to 8 times with each foot.

HIP ROTATION SEQUENCE FOR FEET AND ANKLES

Gently rotating the leg within the hip socket loosens congealed tissue that tends to glue the hips and make them feel tight and stiff. This is a feel-good exercise!

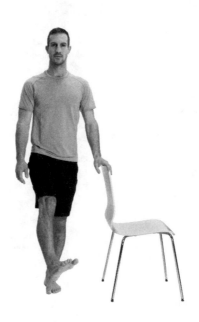

1. Stand with your chair to one side, holding on to it with one or both hands.

2. Lift the opposite leg with the foot flexed. Keep your standing leg slightly bent.

3. Slowly rotate your extended leg within the hip socket, in one direction and then in the other, being sure to isolate the leg from the hip. (Do not let your hip move while you rotate your leg.)

4. Rotate your leg in as far as you can, then hold it. Then try to rotate the leg a little farther. Again, hold it.

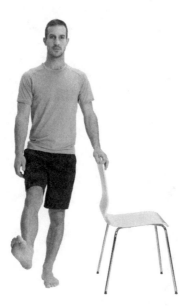

5. Take a deep breath and then rotate your leg in the other direction.

6. Repeat 4 times on both legs.

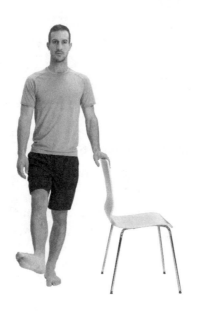

SHIN, CALF, ANKLE, AND FOOT MOBILITY SEQUENCE: LEVEL 1

Doing this heel raiser with a plié is a really powerful way to instantly relieve foot, calf, and shin pain by simultaneously stretching and strengthening the entire lower leg and foot. Take your time and slowly build your strength and flexibility until you can comfortably do a maximum of 6 repetitions. Never do more than 6 in one workout.

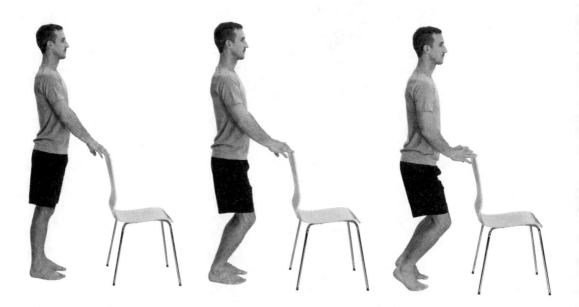

1. Face your chair and hold the back of it with both hands. Stand close enough to the chair that your elbows can remain slightly bent.

2. Slowly bend your knees so that you can feel your muscles stretching (a movement known in ballet as a plié).

3. Then slowly raise your heels so you can feel your muscles doing the work of lifting your entire body weight. (Keep your movements slow; quick movements prevent the strengthening benefits.)

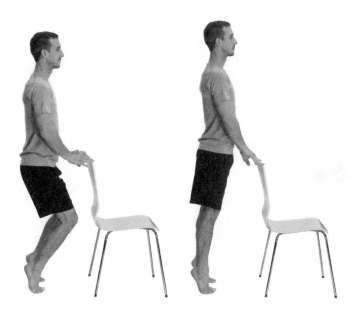

4. With your heels still raised as high as possible, *slowly* straighten your legs. (The slow speed will actively stretch the shins, helping relieve your pain.)

5. Slowly lower your heels until you are standing flat on your feet in the starting position.

6. Repeat the entire exercise 3 to 6 times.

SHIN, CALF, ANKLE, AND FOOT MOBILITY SEQUENCE: LEVEL 2

Level 2 of the shin, calf, ankle, and foot sequence is done in a wider stance. The wider stance increases the degree of pull on the shin muscles. This is to be done after completing Level 1, in the narrower stance. Don't skip to Level 2, as these two exercises are meant to be done in sequence, Level 1 then 2, to prepare the muscles for this deep stretch.

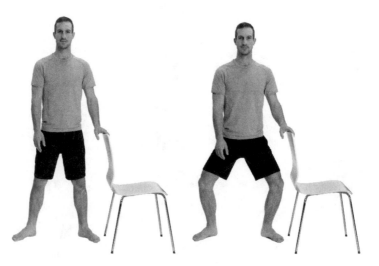

1. Hold on to the back of your chair with one hand. Begin in a wide stance, with your feet slightly turned out. You can stand beside or behind your chair, wherever you feel most secure.

2. Slowly bend your knees, making sure that the thighs are in line with the feet and not dropping in front of the knees.

3. Slowly raise your heels. (You probably will feel a strong tug on your shin muscles. This is good, as you are stretching your tight muscles.)

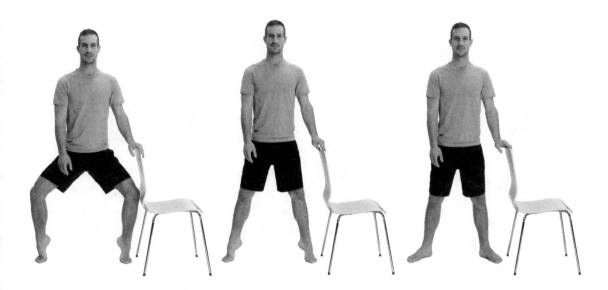

4. With your heels still raised as high as possible, *slowly* straighten your legs. The slow speed will safely stretch the shins, helping relieve the pain of tight shins.

5. Slowly lower your heels to the ground until you are standing flat on your feet in the starting position. (The slow tempo will strengthen all the muscles of your feet, right up the leg into your hips.)

6. Repeat 3 or 4 times.

ANKLE EXERCISE

This exercise is designed to strengthen the ankle, feet, and toe bones, as well as strengthen and increase the flexibility of the muscles of the lower limbs. Your ankles and knees support the weight of your entire body throughout this exercise, so protecting them with clean alignment is essential.

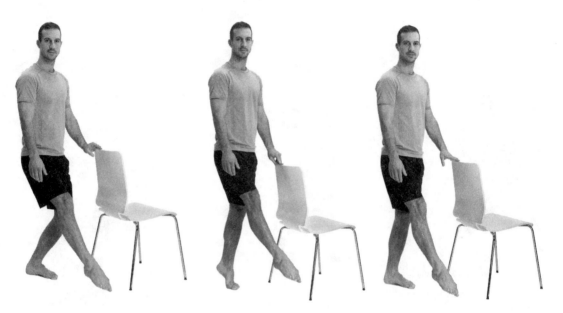

1. Stand with your chair to one side, holding on to it with one hand. Extend your opposite leg to the front, keeping your standing leg slightly bent.

2. Keep your back straight.

3. Slowly straighten your standing leg, and once the leg is fully straightened, lift that heel slowly.

4. Slowly lower your heel and bend your knee to return to your starting position.

5. Repeat 4 to 8 times per leg.

Incorrect Posture in Ankle Strengthening Exercise

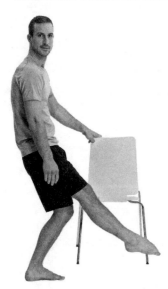

Do not tuck your tailbone or round your spine in the ankle-strengthening exercise. This places stress on your knees and creates an imbalance in your hip flexor muscles, leading to knee and back pain.

CALF SEQUENCE FOR FEET AND ANKLES

This exercise will stretch and strengthen the muscles and tendons of the calf—the Achilles tendon and the soleus and gastrocnemius muscles—which must be stretched simultaneously. If you stretch only one of the two calf muscles, you will cause an imbalance in your calves, leading to discomfort, pain, or injury. Actually, it's very common for people to stretch only one muscle in this group, as most are unaware we have two separate muscles in the calf that must be stretched equally.

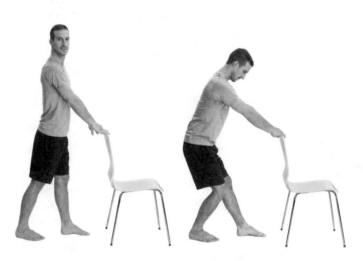

1. Hold the back of your chair with both hands. Stand with one foot slightly in front the other.

2. Slowly bend your back knee while pressing your back heel into the floor. You will feel a stretch in your Achilles tendon (which is part of your calf muscle group).

3. Hold this stretch for 6 seconds to allow your muscles to release into a deeper stretch.

4. Shift your weight onto your front leg, while bending your front knee.

5. Straighten your back leg and lift your back heel off the floor while keeping your toes flexed on the floor.

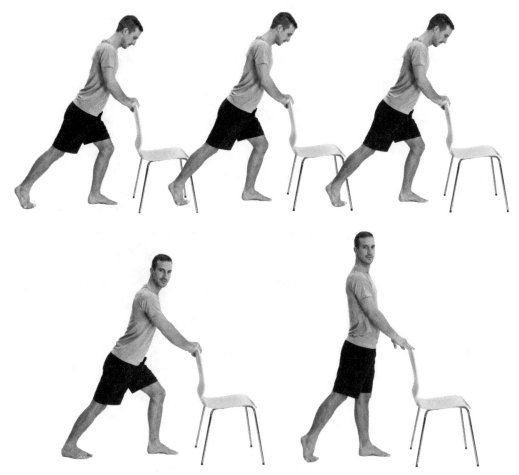

6. Slowly try to press your back heel into the floor; you will feel a deep stretch in the calf.

7. Keeping your weight on your bent front leg, lift and slowly lower your heel until it touches the ground. With each lifting and lowering of your heel, you will feel a deeper calf stretch. Hold the lower phase for 6 seconds.

8. Repeat the entire sequence, from top to bottom, 3 times slowly on each leg.

SQUASH LUNGES

This exercise will lengthen and strengthen the muscles around your knees, decompressing the joint and helping relieve knee pain.

1. Hold the back of your chair with both hands. Place your feet close together and bend your knees.

2. Rapidly kick one leg sideways while simultaneously and rapidly straightening the standing leg.

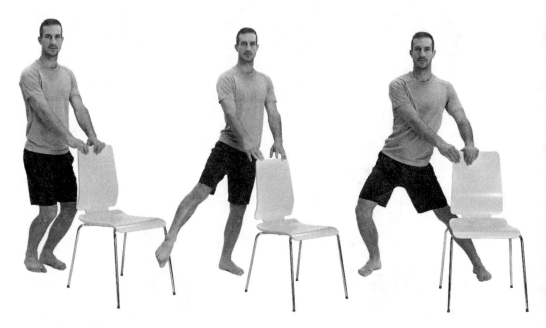

3. Point the foot of the extended leg.

4. Slowly land on your extended leg in a controlled fall. To control your fall, tighten the muscles around your knees and pull your torso upward out of your hips. (The controlled fall is the secret to strengthening your muscles and protecting your knees.)

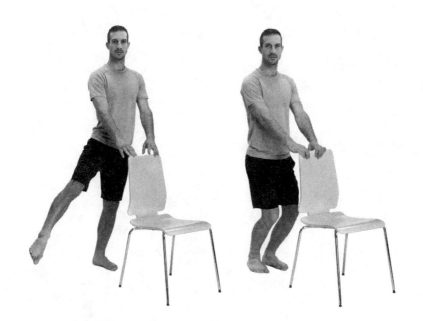

5. Push yourself upright to return to the standing leg.

CHAPTER 7

The Knee Workout

An analytical man by nature and profession, Greg McKenney, a San Francisco accountant, has calculated how much money he saved because of his decision to do the Essentrics program every day: $30,000.

That's the amount of revenue the self-employed accounting consultant figures he would have lost had he undergone two operations recommended by his doctors to end his knee pain. The first involved the surgical breaking of his tibia (shinbone) to correct a slightly bowed left leg, and a second to rebuild the damaged cartilage of his left knee.

But after discovering *Classical Stretch* on his local PBS station, Greg avoided both surgeries and a long, problematic recovery. "Now I have my life back and 22 minutes of joyful exercise every day was the 'investment' that it took. Miranda, I'm your biggest fan," Greg wrote in a 2015 email. "I shudder to think what my life would have been like if I hadn't found *Classical Stretch*."

For fifty-one-year-old Greg, exercise had always energized his life and kept him physically and mentally healthy. As a former cruise ship fitness director, he derives joy from movement, especially windsurfing and kite surfing. Most recently, he has become enamored with kite hydrofoil boards, surfboards that can ride a couple of feet above the water supported by a hydrofoil.

About two years after he began kitesurfing, Greg started experiencing knee pain, a sharp pain—perhaps a 7 on a scale of 10—in an area about the size of a table-tennis ball. Walking downhill or down stairs was especially painful. Greg tracked his pain in his health diary, talked to his doctors, and researched the surgical options they offered. By the spring of 2012, Greg had endured arthroscopic surgeries on both knees. Each operation was carefully scheduled so that postoperative physical therapy would be over and conditioning complete in time for the windsurfing season that runs from mid-March to mid-October in San Francisco, where Greg lives. But late in the summer of 2012, after an extended summer hiking trip, he started experiencing what he described as a severe tightness in his left knee.

His doctors took a closer look at Greg's left leg and determined that it was slightly bowed and was therefore putting a "substantial incorrect weight-bearing" stress on the knee. His leg alignment was off by only 1 or 2 percent, but doctors believed that was enough to put pressure on the medial compartment of his knee. One doctor recommended he wear an offloading brace on that left leg to see whether it would correct the problem. Greg was told that windsurfing would be allowable if he didn't go at it too hard.

The brace did seem to alleviate some pain, but it wasn't comfortable and would slip, requiring adjustments. The major problem, however, was that it increased his risk of deadly injury when he was windsurfing. And by December 2013, Greg was anticipating the osteotomy surgery that would see the surgical breaking of his upper tibia and the careful resetting of the bone into a straighter alignment. To help ensure that the bones knit together in proper alignment, a sophisticated exterior metal frame called a hexapod cage would be connected to the bone by wires or pins to allow for regular adjustments during the recovery period. "I would have been on crutches for four to six weeks and had this metal frame around my leg for four to six months. I would have missed at least eight months of windsurfing and kitesurfing, not to mention the inconvenience," Greg noted.

All of that didn't happen because fate intervened in dramatic fashion just weeks before the scheduled surgery: Greg's appendix burst. It was a hair-raising episode that Greg was fortunate to survive, according to his doctor. After emergency surgery and three nights in the hospital, Greg bounced back to reasonable health. Although his doctors thought he was fit enough for the leg surgery, Greg wanted to regain his full health before submitting to more scalpels and another round of general anesthesia.

And so on January 4, 2013, Greg was lounging on his living room couch, flipping through channels, when he happened to find our program on PBS. "I thought it was so cool . . . and exactly what I needed," he recalled. "I did the workouts every day after that, and in a few days the pain in my knees went away, I kid you not." He stopped wearing the offloading brace, began practicing the workouts regularly, and soon decided that he didn't need the osteotomy surgery. After his introduction to the program, Greg did two workouts every day for some time. Now he does a workout every morning, as well as whenever he feels stiff or his knee tells him he has played too hard.

Severe tightness is caused when the muscles shorten from either extreme concentric strength training or atrophy from a sedentary lifestyle. Obviously in Greg's case it was caused by excessive concentric training of the muscles associated with his tibia (his shins). Every time he landed on his kite board, his muscles would contract to support the impact. This would also explain why walking down stairs or downhill on San Francisco's hilly streets would cause pain. Each downhill step further contracted the already stressed tibia muscles, pulling on the attaching muscles and tendons.

The exercises rebalanced and eccentrically stretched the tibia muscles, lengthening them to relieve the pulling on the knee. When the pulling stopped, the pain disappeared. In addition, the eccentric strengthening benefits offered needed support to Greg's knee, further relieving stress on his knees.

The fact that Greg could enjoy 100 percent relief from his knee pain through correct rebalancing eccentric exercise indicates that the 2 percent bowleggedness was not the cause of the problem. If in fact the bowleggedness was putting "substantial incorrect weight-bearing" on the knee, exercises could not have reversed that. Logic tells me that if the doctors' diagnosis had been correct, Greg's pain would have continued.

We must keep in mind that as advanced as medicine may seem to be, it is a long way from being perfect. Some operations are absolutely necessary to save our lives; however, other surgeries are very much optional. Greg found that correct exercise solved his pain problem, which saved him from the invasiveness of an optional tibia surgery as well as the cost.

As patients, we must use our discretion and look at all the options before deciding whether to have invasive procedures, take potentially addictive drugs, or undergo other measures that may carry significant risks as well as potential benefits.

Greg is a perfect example of injury caused when muscles have been concentrically strengthened and unbalanced. Fortunately, he was young enough that the joint damage was minimal, leaving him pain-free—but only *after* he successfully stretched, strengthened, and rebalanced his legs.

The workout in this chapter is designed for all the many causes of knee pain, from arthritis (one of the leading causes) to injury to recovery from surgery. The exercises will stretch and strengthen the muscles of your feet, ankles, calves, quads, and hips. They are designed to release any tension in the various muscle chains related to the knee pain. Make sure to have a chair nearby for support.

TAI CHI PLIÉ SEQUENCE FOR KNEES

This exercise will stretch and strengthen the quadriceps muscles, decompressing the knees and relieving them from pain.

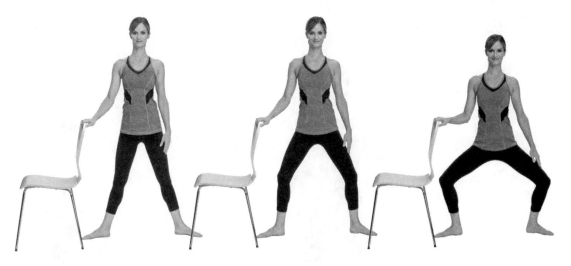

1. Face your chair and hold it with both hands or stand beside it and hold on to it with one hand. Begin in a wide stance.

2. Turn your feet comfortably outward; *never* force the turnout position beyond what is clean alignment as well as feeling comfortable on your knees.

3. Keep your spine straight during the entire tai chi plié sequence.

4. Stand flat on your feet; be aware not to roll your ankles internally or externally.

5. Slowly bend your knees as far as you can, making sure that you remain pain-free.

6. Never go deeper than shown in the photo.

7. Slowly bend your knees, taking about 4 counts to get to your lowest position. Your thighs and knees should always be directly in line with your feet, never dropping in front of them.

8. Once you arrive at your maximum depth of plié, slowly straighten your knees.

9. In each plié, take about 5 seconds to bend your knees and about 5 seconds to straighten your knees.

10. Repeat 8 to 12 pliés.

Correct and Incorrect Feet Positions

These images show various correct and incorrect plié positions. To determine your safe turnout position, slowly turn out your feet until the very last point at which the sole of your foot remains flat on the ground. (If your foot starts to roll forward, you have turned it out too far.)

Correct Feet Positions

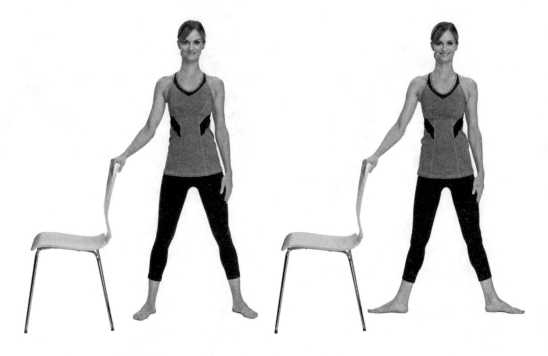

This image shows correct form. It represents someone who has tight hips and cannot turn out her legs farther than this.

This image shows correct form. It represents someone who is very loose and can safely turn out her feet to an extreme degree.

Incorrect Feet Positions

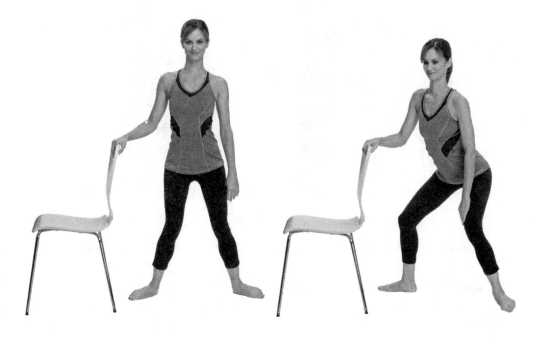

This image shows incorrect form. The feet are rolling forward and the knees are dropping in front of the hips. Allowing your feet to roll forward places dangerous torsion stress on your knees and hips.

This image also shows incorrect form. Allowing your back to tilt forward and your bum to protrude will put stress on your lower vertebrae, knees, and hips.

FOOT SEQUENCE FOR KNEES

This exercise rapidly relieves foot pain by working to release stiffness in the individual articulation of the ankle and toe joints. It will stretch and strengthen the muscles to increase joint flexibility.

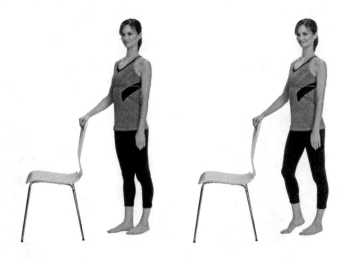

1. Face your chair and hold it with one or both hands. Stand with one foot slightly in front of the other.

2. Slowly lift the heel of the forward foot, shifting your weight forward and pressing your weight onto the ball of your foot. You will feel a deep stretch pulling on your shin muscle.

3. While doing so, make sure your toes stay flat on the ground to increase the flexibility between your toes and the soles of your feet.

4. Maintain clean alignment throughout the movement by keeping your ankle directly over your foot. Never let your ankles roll inward or outward.

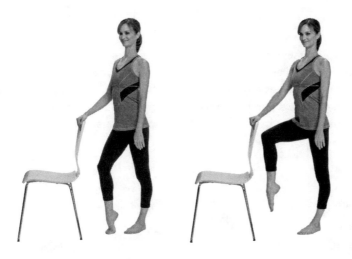

5. Finish the movement by pointing your toes as you lift your foot off the floor.

6. Reverse the steps of the sequence: first lower your toes, then lower your heels.

7. Repeat 4 to 8 times on each foot.

Incorrect Form

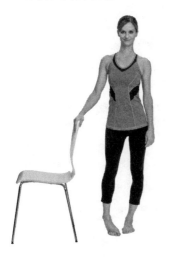

Do not roll your foot out by sickling. *Sickling* is a ballet term for scooping the ankle in such a way that it looks like a farmer's sickle. It is a dangerous misalignment that overstretches the ligaments, weakening the ankle and making it prone to twisting or spraining.

CALF SEQUENCE FOR KNEES

The calf has two equally important muscles: the soleus and the gastrocnemius. They both attach to the Achilles tendon, which attaches to your heel. To prevent injury and relieve pain, the calf muscles must be equally balanced—both muscles must be stretched and strengthened in the same sequence. When you rebalance the calf muscles with this sequence, the pain should go away. The feet and calf muscles directly link to the knees, making these exercises extremely important to relieve knee pain.

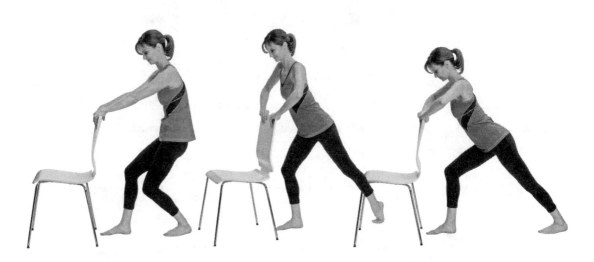

1. Hold the back of your chair with both hands. Place one foot slightly in front of the other.

2. Bend both knees and shift your weight onto the back heel. This will stretch the Achilles tendon and the soleus muscle. Relax into this stretch, letting your weight sink as deeply as possible.

3. Hold the soleus stretch for at least 6 seconds before shifting to the following stretch.

4. Shift your weight onto your front leg, while bending your front knee.

5. Straighten your back leg and lift the back heel off the floor while keeping your toes flexed on the floor.

6. With your weight still on your front leg, straighten the back leg while slowly pressing the back heel into the floor, and lift your bum (see photo). You will feel your large calf muscle (gastrocnemius) stretching. Raise and lower the back heel 3 times slowly.

7. While keeping your weight on your bent front leg, lift and then slowly lower your heel, trying to touch the ground with it. (Your heel might not be able to touch the ground.) With each lifting and lowering of your heel, you should feel a deep toe and calf stretch. Hold the stretch phase for 6 seconds.

8. Repeat the entire sequence from beginning to end 3 times for each leg.

HIP STRETCHING SEQUENCE FOR KNEES

This hip sequence will loosen and stretch a chain of muscles that attaches the torso to the legs. When the hips muscles are tight, the tension in those muscles spirals down into the knees and feet, limiting their movement and leading to pain. The hip joint is a ball-and-socket joint; we do rotational, side-to-side, and forward-and-backward stretches to loosen all parts of the ball and socket. By shifting the thighbone back and forth in the socket during these stretches, you're helping rebalance and loosen any tightness in your hip muscles.

Phase One:

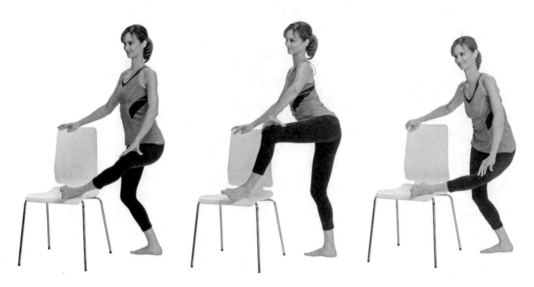

1. Stand diagonally behind your chair and place your outside leg on the seat.

2. Bend both knees while holding the back of the chair for balance.

3. Lift and lower your hips, as though you were swaying your hips side to side.

4. As you sway your hips, you may feel a loosening within your hip socket.

5. Repeat 4 times on each side.

Phase Two:

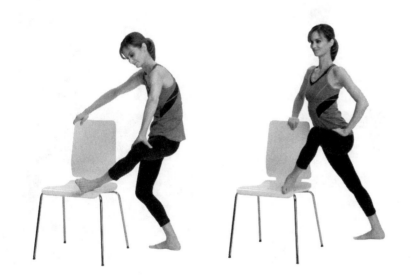

1. Adjust your body to face the seat of the chair for a new series of spine exercises.

2. Start by rounding your spine, dropping your shoulders forward, and tucking your bum under.

3. Slowly shift your spine into the reverse position, arching your back and sticking your bum out while shifting your weight forward. Note: The more you exaggerate the hip shifts, the better the results in loosening the joint.

4. Return to the original position, with your back rounded and your bum tucked under.

5. Repeat the full arching and rounding of the spine sequence 4 times.

PSOAS SEQUENCE FOR KNEES

The psoas muscles (which consist of the psoas major and psoas minor) attach the lower spine to the thighbone. Every time we sit, stand, or walk, we use the psoas muscle group. Because it is used virtually every minute of our waking lives, it tends to get unbalanced, leading to knee injury and pain.

While the psoas is a small muscle group, it's located in an important part of our body: the place where our legs join our torso. When this muscle group becomes either too tight or too weak, it can cause pain downward, affecting the knees, or upward, causing back pain. This exercise will rebalance the psoas muscles, reversing tension and thus relieving pain and discomfort when walking, running, or climbing stairs.

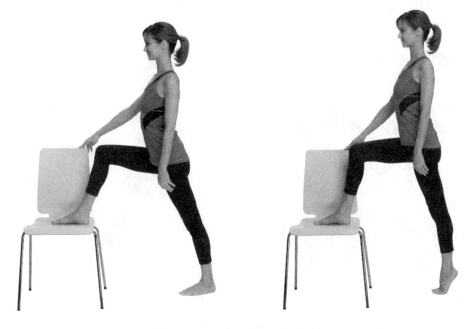

1. Stand beside your chair, and hold the back for support.

2. Place one foot flat on the seat of the chair; your standing leg should be straight and leaning slightly forward.

3. Holding the chair for balance, slowly lift the heel of your standing leg.

4. Bend the knee of your standing leg, and tuck your lower spine (pelvis) under as though you were trying to look at the zipper on your pants. Locking the tucked-under spine,

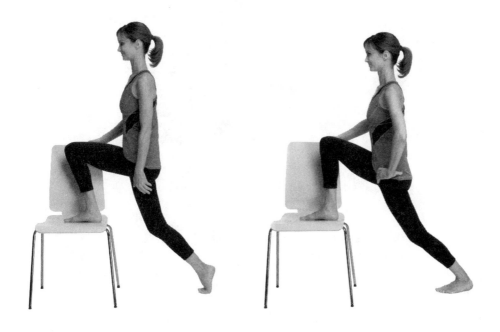

shift your weight forward from your hips toward the chair. It is important to keep your back completely straight.

5. Try to straighten the back leg while pressing the back heel into the floor. Note: Keep your pelvic tuck engaged throughout.

6. Return to the starting position before repeating the entire psoas stretch.

7. Repeat slowly 3 times with each leg.

HAMSTRING FLEXIBILITY SEQUENCE FOR KNEES

Tight hamstrings (a group of muscles that run along the back of the leg from thighbone to knee) restrict the mobility of your hips, knees, and spine. They constantly pull on the knee joint and spinal vertebrae, leading to knee and back pain. In this stretch, we sway the hips and move the bum, creating a self-massage of the hamstrings and hips. The more you move and sway your hips, the faster the muscle of your hamstrings will release tension and permit you to go into a deep stretch.

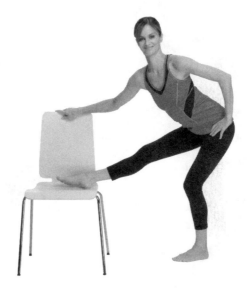

1. Stand beside your chair, with one leg resting on the seat and the standing leg slightly bent. Hold the back of the chair for balance.

2. Try to straighten the leg on the chair. Note: If you have tight hamstrings you may not be able to straighten your knee. Don't worry if you can't completely straighten it— many people can't!

3. Keeping your spine as straight as possible, bend forward over the lifted leg. Note: It is better not to bend too far forward, as you will lose some of the stretch the moment your spine rounds.

4. Arch your back, pushing your bum toward the opposite end of the room; you should feel a deep hamstring stretch.

5. Slowly lift and lower your hips in a gently swaying motion. At the same time, reach your arm directly over your leg.

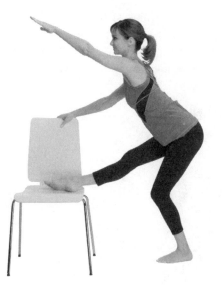

6. Repeat at least 4 times with each leg, spending between 2 and 3 minutes on each leg.

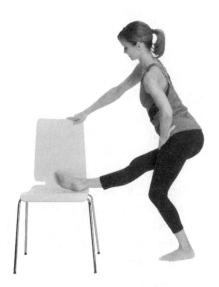

QUADRICEPS STRETCH FOR KNEES

The quadriceps are four large muscles at the front of your thigh that cross over your knee joint. When your quadriceps are tight, they will squeeze the knee joint, leading to compression, loss of range of motion, and pain. Doing these exercise will release the compression on the knees and help you regain full and safe range of motion.

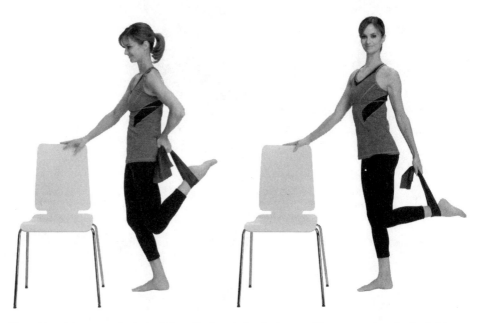

1. Stand beside your chair, holding the back for balance. Keep your back straight.

2. Tuck your hips under while bending your standing leg,

3. Raise your outside leg and, with your hand on your ankle, slowly pull your ankle toward your bum. If you have trouble reaching your ankle, use a stretch band or small towel to comfortably pull your ankle (as shown in the photo). This will permit you to keep your back straight during this sequence.

4. When your muscles won't stretch any more, gently release your leg; no stretch should last longer than 5 seconds. Note: As you are pulling in a stretch, you will feel the muscles slowly relaxing and releasing into the stretch. At the point they stop releasing, shift into the next movement. Holding beyond that point can be counterproductive and may actually tighten your muscles.

5. Repeat the stretch 3 times with each leg.

Incorrect Quadriceps Stretch

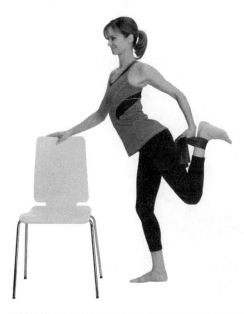

Do not arch your back or raise your bum. A raised bum will release the stretch and nullify the benefits of this sequence.

IT BAND ROTATION

The iliotibial (IT) band is a band of fibrous tissue that runs down the outside of the thigh. Its main purpose is to support and stabilize the knee joint to stop your knee from wobbling sideways. When the IT band becomes tight, it can pull the knee joint out of alignment and cause damage and pain to the knee. Note: When you reach your maximum IT band stretch, you will likely feel an "ouch" sensation. This is one occasion when a tiny bit of discomfort is okay in exercise.

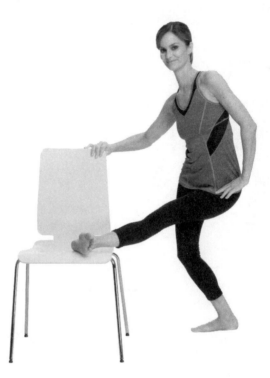

1. Stand beside your chair with your outside leg resting on the seat. Hold the chair with your opposite hand for balance. Flex the foot on the chair, and bend *only* your standing knee.

2. Slowly drop the hip of your raised leg, while rotating it outward. Try to rotate your leg so much that the top of the flexed foot will touch the chair. (That's impossible to do, but keeping this image in your head will help you stretch in the right direction.)

3. You will feel an uncomfortable stretch in one of two places: your hip or your knee.

4. Rotate your leg slowly as you lift and drop your hip into and out of the stretch. Note: This stretch usually hurts a little because you are actually stretching tendons as well as muscles. Tendons are full of nerve endings, which make them super-sensitive. Moving slowly will guarantee that you do not damage the tendons during this stretch. Do not stop stretching when you feel the discomfort but continue to move slowly and carefully. The discomfort you feel comes from the tendon being pulled but should never result in a sensation of pain.

5. Release the stretch, returning to your starting position.

6. Repeat the stretch 3 times on each leg.

LONG ADDUCTOR STRETCH

To rebalance your full hip region, you must stretch and strengthen the muscles at the front, outside, back, and inside of your leg. When the long adductor muscles of the hip (your inner thigh muscles) are tight and stiff, they pull on the inside of the knee, leading to injury and pain. This exercise targets those specific muscles.

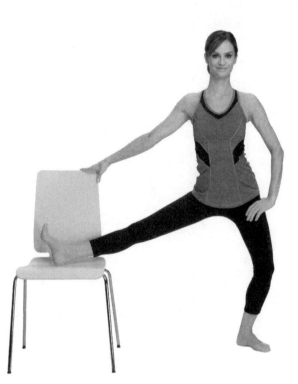

1. Stand next to your chair, facing the front, and rest the leg nearest the chair on the seat. Flex your foot.

2. Bend your standing leg and *try* to straighten the leg on the chair.

3. Bend forward while rotating the leg on the chair toward the front of the room. Keep your spine straight, and let your bum stick out behind.

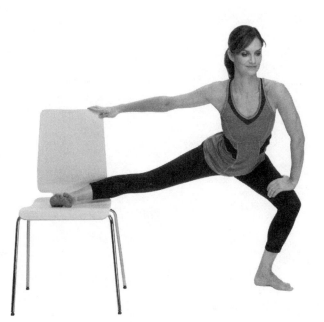

4. Play with this stretch by slowly bending forward and rotating the extended leg in the hip socket and then returning to a straighter position. Note: Go gently and try to find the place that best stretches your inner thigh muscles. Everyone feels this stretch in a slightly different place. Never force this stretch to go too deep; there are sensitive ligaments involved that you don't want to overstretch.

5. Take about 6 seconds for each leg rotation and bend forward.

6. Repeat at least 3 times on each side.

CHAPTER 8

The Hip Workout

W hen Anik Bissonnette danced, ballet audiences worldwide were capti- vated by her grace and classical line. Critics struggled to find adjectives laudatory enough to describe her performances.

The principal dancer with Les Grands Ballets Canadiens, an acclaimed company in Montreal, Anik was a regular guest artist with many of the world's greatest companies, among them the Paris Opera. She performed lead roles in *Swan Lake*, *Giselle*, *Romeo and Juliet*, and *Cinderella*, but in 2004, after twenty-four years of performing, Anik suffered a hip injury that put her career in jeopardy.

"I had a microtear of the labrum," recalled Anik, referring to the acetabular labrum, a fibrous rim of cartilage around the hip socket that is important in the normal function of the hip. It helps keep the head of the femur inside the acetabulum (hip socket) and provides stability to the joint.

The pain from this injury prevented Anik from extending her leg to the side as high as she wanted to. In order to relieve the pain and get her leg up, she slightly readjusted the alignment of her body. Dancers do this all the time when they have injuries; it's known as cheating. It helps them look like they are doing the movement correctly—but they aren't, and their bodies know it. The result for Anik was a cascade of new aches and pains, nota- bly in the back muscles—a potentially career-ending situation for the ballerina.

Her doctors ruled out surgery because the labral tear was so small. Even if the micro- tear had been operable, Anik would have required months, if not years, to recover enough to return to the extreme demands of her profession. And it was time she didn't have. At forty-two, Anik was already a decade past the average age of retirement for ballerinas. The average dancer leaves the stage before age thirty-four, and more than 35 percent cite physical injuries as the culprit. Many of those young retirees also have to deal with the psychological pain of leaving their dream profession and letting go of hard-won achievements that required years of demanding training, followed by intense competition to land a job.

Yet the pain from the injury was making it impossible for Anik to participate in the daily ballet class that dancers use to keep in shape. Without the daily ballet class, she would fall rapidly out of shape, a situation that would itself end her career.

As the principal dancer of Les Grands Ballet Canadiens, Anik had ready access to an array of specialized health-care professionals, but she couldn't find relief from the hip pain. "I was always in physiotherapy," she recalled. To save her career, Anik went on a quest to find a pain-free workout program to replace the daily dance class. She tried programs such as yoga and Pilates, but they didn't give her the strength and stamina she required, nor did they relieve her of pain. (And she found them very boring!)

Anik was still searching for a suitable workout when—by happy coincidence—I reached out to her to see if she'd be interested in starring in my Essentrics DVDs for the French-speaking market. Anik says the memory of her first class with us was still fresh in her mind, more than a decade later. "It was as though I did a complete (technical) ballet class. It was as intense as that for me," she said. "The program is so well conceived that there was no movement that caused me pain, and there was no movement I was unable to do because of pain."

When she left for Mexico to film with us, she worried that the two-week trip would see her return lightly tanned but not in the tip-top shape required to begin rehearsals for her next leading role. *Au contraire!* When she returned from the two weeks of exclusive Essentrics workouts, she was stronger and in better shape than she had been before leaving. And, best of all, she was no longer in pain. Not only had she spent several hours doing Essentrics every day, we'd also spent hours discussing anatomy and how through correct training the human body can remain pain-free and heal itself. Anik said it gave her a new appreciation of how her body worked.

"I was really, really surprised that when I came back to Montreal, I was in so much better shape than when I had left," Anik recalled. "I had strengthened the muscles around my hips, which was so important to do. When you have an injury, you want to make those muscles move and have the blood circulating to help heal the injury." The boot-camp experience of two solid weeks of Essentrics put her on a new path, one that she credits with adding years to her career.

In just two weeks, Anik was able to rebalance all of the muscles that the injury had unbalanced. Rebalancing her body's muscles readjusted her hip alignment, making her stronger overall. As a consequence of this realignment and rebalancing, all the pain she had been suffering from, including the hip pain, disappeared.

Anik used Essentrics as her only workout program during the rest of her dance career. "I would say it added a good five years to my career," she estimated, "because I was in such good shape and pain-free." Of her last performance as the principal dancer with Les Grands Ballets in June 2007, critics wrote that her performance "showed her still in excellent form" with a "silhouette hardly changed" from her teenage years. In 2009, a few weeks before celebrating her forty-seventh birthday, Anik retired as a ballerina.

When we are in pain, like Anik, we instinctively adjust our bodies so as not to stress the source of the pain. For Anik, it was her hip. She instinctively adjusted her leg alignment to take the pressure off of her hip, where she was suffering from a labrum tear. Protecting an injury can cause us to develop a limp. The limp, in turn, leads to a chain reaction of imbalances throughout our entire body, which often leads to other injuries and more pain. An injury that starts off as hip pain in our twenties might spiral into chronic back pain decades later. This is precisely what happened to Anik, but her pain disappeared when she rebalanced her full body.

Anik was surprised that relatively easy workouts could make her chronic hip and back pain disappear. Still, Essentrics didn't heal her torn labrum, as labrum tissue cannot be healed through exercise—it requires the skilled hand of a surgeon. But we did rebalance the muscles around Anik's hip. The exercises rotated, stretched, and strengthened her muscles in and around the socket and thus relieved the pressure and stress on the tear.

Anik's brain registered that the danger was gone, so it turned off the pain signal and Anik felt as though the injury had healed. In fact, the tear was still there, but the labrum was now protected.

These exercises, done for 30 minutes a day, will reverse atrophy, weakness, and pain in hips and groin muscles. Make sure to have a chair nearby for support.

SIMPLE TAI CHI PLIÉ FOR HIPS

Tai chi pliés are exercises that stretch and strengthen the quadriceps and gluteus muscles, removing the excessive tugging on the hips and joints to relieve pain rapidly. They strengthen the muscles in a lengthened position, liberating and energizing all the surrounding joints.

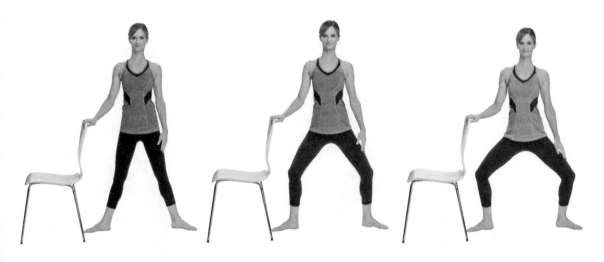

1. Begin by standing in a comfortably wide stance. Hold the chair with one hand. Note: You can also face the chair and hold it with both hands if that helps you feel more secure and balanced.

2. Turn your feet out in a wide tai chi stance; this will help you do the plié with your knees in line over your feet (not dropping in front of your feet).

3. Be careful not to roll your ankles forward or backward.

4. Keep your spine straight during the entire sequence; don't bend forward and let your bum protrude as you would in a squat.

5. Slowly bend your knees and plié as deeply as you can while still remaining pain-free. (Do not go deeper than knee height.)

6. Count to 5 as you bend your knees. Then count to 5 again as you straighten them.

7. Repeat 4 to 8 pliés.

TAI CHI PLIÉ WITH HIP SWING

In this exercise, you will repeat the same directions as in the simple tai chi plié but add a hip swing at the bottom of the plié. The swing of the hips will stretch one side of the hips (gluteus) and then the other. This swing loosens tight hips—and feels really good as you are doing it!

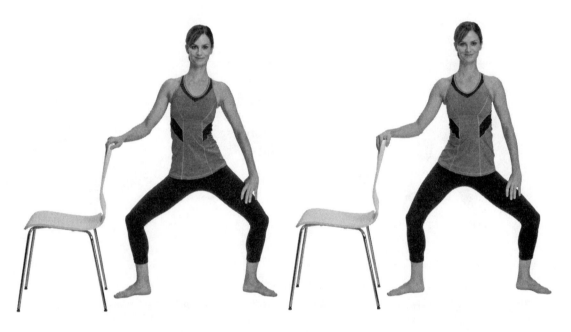

1. Repeat the directions in the simple tai chi plié until you get to the bottom of the plié. Remain at the bottom of the plié to do 8 slow hip swings before straightening your legs.

2. At the bottom of the plié, slowly swing your hips from side to side, one hip at a time, trying to swing as far as you can into each hip.

3. You should feel a stretch in your bum, inner leg, or groin.

4. Repeat the full plié 2 to 4 times, swinging your hips 8 times within each plié.

SWINGS

The purpose of swings is to remove dead tissue and congealed fluids that can cause stickiness and a sensation of immobility in the hip joints. A glued hip joint has lost its natural range of motion, causing the surrounding muscles to atrophy. Immobility almost always leads to pain. Try to perform these exercises with a smooth, fluid motion, never stopping to hold a position.

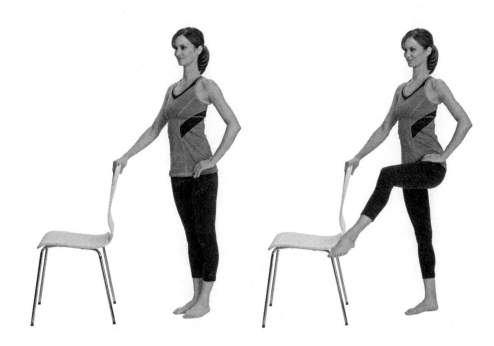

1. Stand beside your chair, with both feet together. Hold the chair with one hand and place your other hand on your hip.

2. Before starting, take a moment to relax your hips. Keep your back straight throughout the exercise, and don't let your body rock back and forth as you swing your legs.

3. In a smooth and fluid motion, slightly bend the outside leg and swing it front to back like the pendulum of a clock.

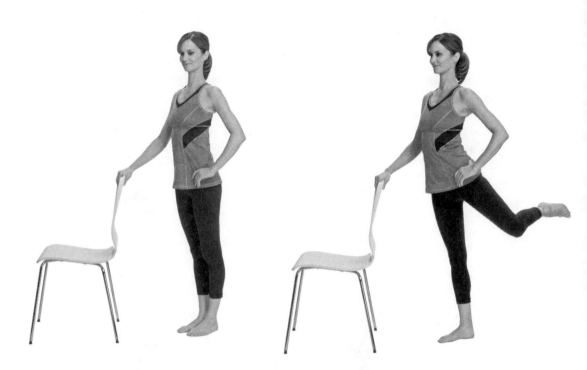

4. Keep your leg low; focus on maintaining an easy, relaxed swinging motion. Note: You can choose to turn your knee out to the side a little bit, or not—go according to your own comfort level.

5. Don't stop to hold the knee at the front or back, just maintain constant motion and keep swinging throughout the exercise.

6. Repeat 16 to 32 swings per leg.

HIP CLEANERS

Hip cleaners are similar to swings in that they work at sloughing away the congealed connective tissue that collects in the hip socket and creates immobility, leading to loss of range of motion and hip pain. Remember, the hip is a ball-and-socket joint. These hip cleaners roll the ball part around in every part of the socket, acting like a gentle scouring pad to clean debris glued in the socket. They also loosen every muscle that attaches the ball-and-socket joint together. Hip cleaners are another feel-good exercise; athletes tend to do these repetitively because they feel so good.

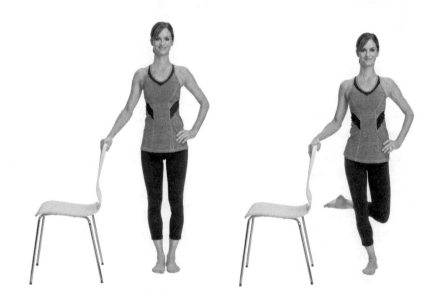

1. Begin by standing with your feet parallel, steadying yourself on the back of your chair.

2. Slightly bend the knee on the leg closest to the chair, lift the other foot, and place it diagonally behind you while bending the knee on that leg.

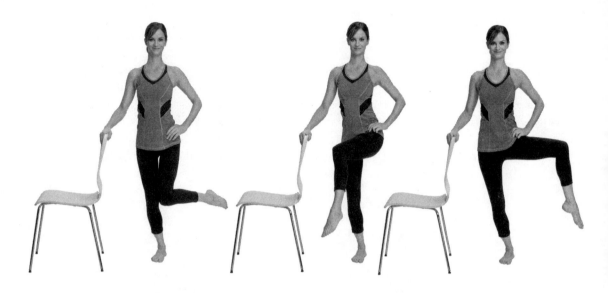

3. Rotate the thigh on your outside leg internally in the hip socket; you will notice that the foot will automatically swing to the outside.

4. Draw your knee diagonally across the front of your body; you will feel a stretch in your bum. Note: While doing this exercise, hold your hips still as you rotate the leg within the hip socket.

5. Lift the bent leg higher and draw it across the front of the body, opening your hip. Finish with your leg spread out as wide open to the side as possible.

6. Return to the starting position.

7. Repeat 4 to 8 times per leg.

PSOAS SEQUENCE FOR HIPS

The psoas muscles attach in the front of your thighbone and finish in several of the lower vertebra, or lumbar spine. Due to poor walking or lifestyle habits, the psoas tends to tighten and shrink, unbalancing the entire hip region and leading to chronic hip pain. A tight psoas is common in people over forty.

This exercise will stretch the psoas muscles, relieving hip tension and the resulting back pain. When the psoas muscles are healthy and well stretched, you'll have greater ease of movement when walking, running, and climbing the stairs.

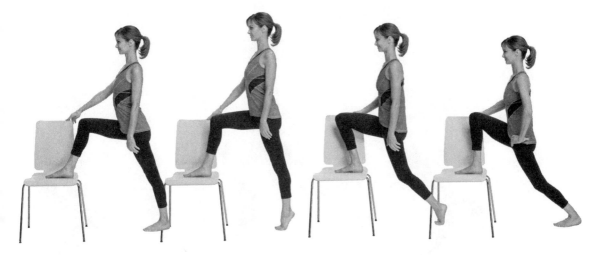

1. Stand beside your chair. Place one foot flat on the seat of the chair with your knee bent and the other leg straight behind you. Note: Don't stand too close to the chair.

2. Holding the back of the chair for support, raise the heel of your standing leg.

3. Bend the knee of your standing leg, and tuck your bum under your hips while shifting your weight forward, toward the seat of the chair.

4. Try to lock your bum in the tucked-under position while simultaneously trying to straighten the back leg and press the back heel into the floor. (You probably won't be able to put your back heel on the floor if you lock your bum in the tucked-under position. That's okay!) You will most likely feel a stretch somewhere in your thigh; everyone feels the stretch in a different place.

5. Return to the starting position.

6. Repeat the psoas stretch very slowly 3 times on each leg.

HIP REBALANCING SEQUENCE

The tension in tight hip muscles limits range of motion and blocks comfortable movement; walking, running, sitting, and even standing become painful. Your hips are attached to your spine and thighbone, so in this sequence, you will be simultaneously doing spine and hamstring stretches. The hip sequence will loosen and stretch a chain of muscles that attach your torso to your legs.

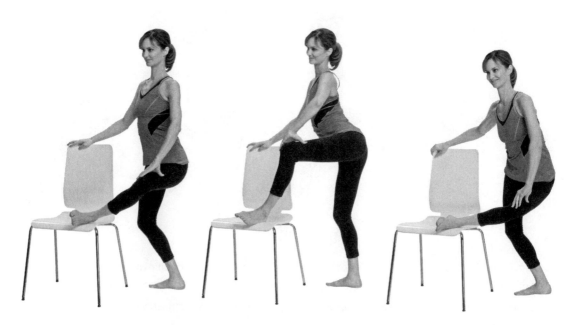

1. Stand diagonally behind your chair and place the outside leg on the seat of the chair.
2. Bend both knees while holding the back of the chair for balance.
3. Lift and lower your hips as though you were swaying your hips side to side.
4. As you sway your hips, you may feel a loosening within your hip socket.
5. Repeat 4 times.

6. Change your spine's position for a new series of spine exercises.

7. Start by rounding your spine, dropping your shoulders forward, and tucking your bum under.

8. Slowly shift your spine into the reverse position, arching your back and sticking your bum out while shifting your weight forward. Note: The more you exaggerate the hip shifts, the better the results in loosening the joint. This sequence shifts the thighbone back and forth in the socket during these stretches, helping rebalance and loosen any tightness in the hip muscles.

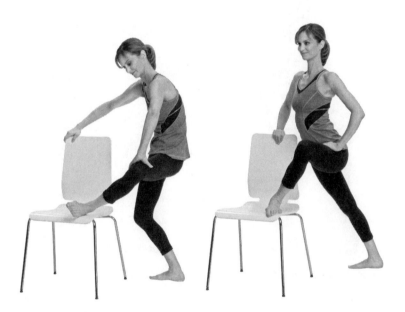

9. Return to the original position, with your back rounded and your bum tucked under.

10. Repeat the full arching and rounding of the spine sequence 4 times.

QUADRICEPS STRETCH FOR HIPS

The quadriceps are four large muscles at the front of your thigh that cross over your knee joint. When your quadriceps are tight, they will squeeze the knee joint, leading to compression, loss of range of motion, and pain. Doing these exercise will liberate the compression on the knees and help you regain full and safe range of motion.

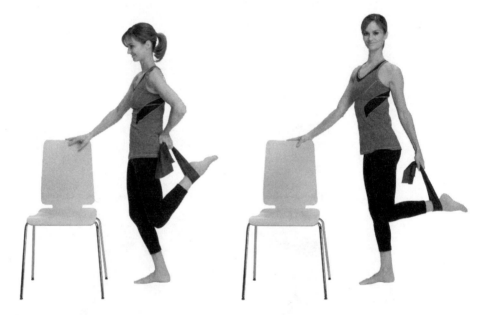

1. Stand next to your chair, holding the back for balance. Keep your back straight.

2. Tuck your hips under while bending your standing leg.

3. Raise your outside leg and, with your hand on your ankle, slowly pull your ankle toward your bum. If you have trouble reaching your ankle, use a stretch band or a small towel to comfortably pull your ankle (as shown in the photo). This will permit you to keep your back straight during this sequence.

4. When your muscles won't stretch any more gently, release your leg; no stretch should last longer than 5 seconds. Note: As you are pulling in a stretch, you will feel the muscles slowly relaxing and releasing into the stretch. At the point they stop releasing, shift into the next movement. Holding beyond that point can be counterproductive and actually tighten your muscles.

5. Repeat the stretch 3 times with each leg.

HIP-BLAST SEQUENCE

This hip-blast sequence employs a neurological technique called proprioceptive neuro-muscular facilitation (PNF). As you do this exercise, you will contract the muscle; release the contraction; relax more; and then, finally, stretch. This PNF technique will give you an amazing feeling of freedom in your hips. This hip blast is a favorite of athletes, like runners, who often suffer from tight hips.

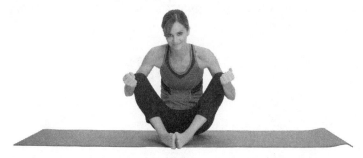

1. Sit on the ground with your knees bent and the soles of your feet touching comfortably in front of you.

2. Lift your knees and hold them tightly with your arms, and then try to force your knees toward the floor. The trick here is to block your knees from lowering; this will create a buildup of tension in the groin (or hip region, depending on the person).

3. Let go of your knees, and try to relax the hips and groin for 2 or 3 seconds.

4. Hold your shins just above your ankles, and place your elbows on your knees.

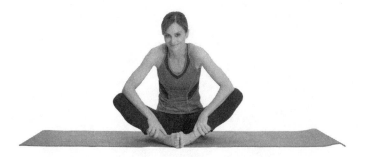

5. Bend forward, using your elbows to push down on your knees; you will feel a strong stretch in your groin or hips.

6. Slowly repeat the full sequence 3 to 4 times.

HIP AND GROIN STRETCH

This old-school gym favorite, done the Essentrics way, is great for targeting and lengthening shortened groin muscles. Doing this stretch every day will also further help open and relieve pressure on your hip joints.

1. Sit comfortably (your back can be rounded), holding your shins just above your ankles.

2. Place one elbow on one knee and gently press down on the knee; you will feel a stretch in one groin muscle.

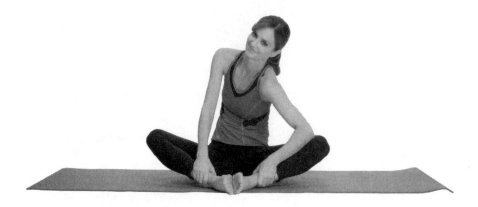

3. Hold for about 6 seconds.

4. Change to the other knee, and stretch the other groin muscle.

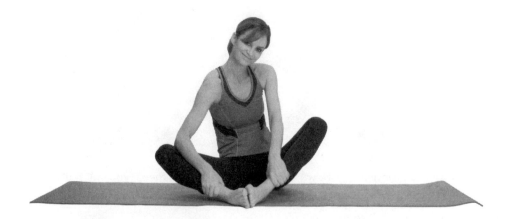

5. Repeat 4 times, alternating sides each time.

6. Add on a deeper stretch by placing both hands on either knee and gently pressing down on the knee. Hold this deep stretch for 6 seconds and release the pressure.

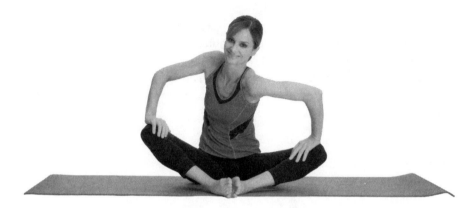

7. Repeat 4 times, alternating sides each time.

PNF CHEAT SHEET

Remember, proprioceptive neuromuscular facilitation (PNF) is a technique used primarily by physiotherapists to safely and rapidly increase flexibility. The principles of PNF will be extremely useful to you in these hip sequences. For a detailed discussion of PNF, turn to page 55. But for now, here's an overview:

- Contract your muscles.
- Hold the contraction for 3 to 6 seconds.
- Relax all of your muscles.
- Relax even deeper and wiggle to release all tension.
- Push the newly relaxed muscles to stretch them.

HAMSTRING STRETCH FOR HIPS

The hamstring muscle crosses two joints; it starts on your hipbone and finishes by attaching to your shinbone. The hamstring—located on the back side of the leg, opposite from the quadriceps—is one of the largest muscle groups in the body. When it is tight and stiff, it pulls the hipbone close to the thighbone, squeezing the joint and causing joint compression. We lose our range of motion—and walking, running, and even sitting can become painful and difficult. (Even getting on and off a toilet can become a problem!) This PNF hamstring stretch will loosen the tension, decompressing the joint and relieving hip pain.

1. Lie on your back, with your spine and hips flat on the ground.

2. Bend one leg, keeping the foot of that leg flat on the ground.

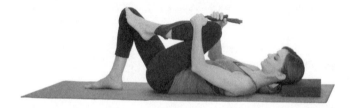

3. Raise the other leg, bending the knee of that leg. Hold the knee with both hands and pull it toward your chest.

4. While doing this, relax your bum and wiggle it under you. (Wiggling your bum will force your hip muscle to relax, making the next movement easier to do.)

5. Release your hold on the knee, raise your leg higher, and try to straighten the knee. Note: If your hamstrings are tight, you may not be able to straighten your knee completely; in that case, leave it slightly bent.

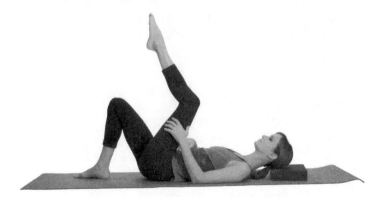

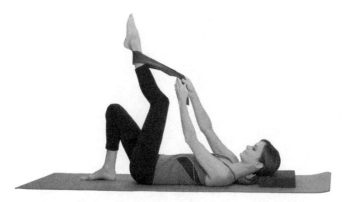

6. Wrap a stretch band comfortably around your lower leg, near your ankle. Use the band to pull your leg toward your chest while keeping your head flat on the floor.

7. Using the PNF techniques (see box), resist with a push, release, relax more with the wiggle, and then pull again.

8. Push against the band, trying to lower your leg toward the floor. (The band will stop you from being able to lower your leg too far.) Push for 3 to 6 seconds.

9. Stop pushing against the band and relax your hips for 3 seconds.

10. Wiggle your bum for 3 seconds.

11. Using the band, pull your leg toward your chest again. (The band will help you deepen your stretch.) Hold for about 6 seconds.

12. Relax 6 seconds before starting again.

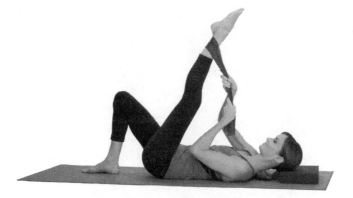

13. Repeat 3 times before changing legs.

CHAPTER 9

The Back Workout

D r. Sharon Cadiz is a retired director of the Clinical Consultation Program at the City of New York's Administration for Children's Services. At age sixty-three, she's still active, working as a consultant and riding her bicycle to a shared office in her neighborhood. But despite her active lifestyle, Sharon struggles daily with back pain.

Sharon's history with back pain dates to early childhood. She remembers pain radiating from her legs to her lower back when she was just eight years old. At fifteen, she suffered a bad fall that left her with a great deal of neck pain. Sharon links that accident to the chronic back pain that continues to persist decades later.

As an adult, she was diagnosed with degenerative disc disease, and in her late forties she suffered a painful two-year bout with sciatica. Sharon also believes that the stress and tension of a demanding career contributed to her backaches throughout her working years.

Always a believer that exercise and time in the gym could remedy anything, she embraced an intense fitness schedule to offset stress and weight gain. After doing three to five workouts a week at the local gym for years, she was stopped short by pain. After her fifty-second birthday, she was taking a step class in the gym and felt an explosive pain in her right calf. "For some unknown reason, I kept going, even though the flash of pain was like what I would imagine a gunshot wound would feel like," she recalled. "Within a matter of days, I was in excruciating pain." Her chronic back pain was now accompanied by severe leg pain.

Several days later, she finally saw her doctor, who gave her a shot of cortisone and a prescription for pain medication. The pain left her incapacitated, forcing her to work from home. She was in too much pain to walk, let alone commute to work. "I spent a lot of time in the recliner during the day. My nighttime sleep was very brief, a little sleep here and there," she said. "I've given birth twice and gone through a variety of injuries in my life, but I've never known pain like that."

From March to June, she subsisted on the medication that doctors prescribed for back pain and sleeping. However, the medication did not take the pain away during those months at home—all it did was take the edge off a little bit. "That's how extreme the pain was," she said.

Her doctors concluded that her best option to relieve the back pain, which was caused by a herniated disc, was lumbar laminectomy surgery. While still housebound prior to the surgery, Sharon was flipping through channels on the television when she came across *Classical Stretch* on PBS. "As I watched," she said, "I was drawn to mimic some of the movements and suddenly found myself seated on the floor fully engaged in the program. I felt relief immediately."

In June 2004, Sharon underwent the lumbar laminectomy surgery. "I was pain-free for the most part, but I had a new problem, called 'drop foot,'" Sharon recalled. "Nobody could help me with it. Nobody."

Drop foot is a term used to describe a limp foot that seems to hang half lifeless at the end of the leg. The foot has no strength to support balance, making walking unstable and falls common. This neurological condition causes muscular and anatomical damage. People with drop foot often support their ankle with a brace to prevent the foot from flopping.

The previous months of bed rest prior to the surgery had left Sharon's muscles too weak to move her injured leg. This forced her to swing her leg with each step, compounding the tripping and falling from drop foot. Postsurgery, Sharon had regular physiotherapy sessions, but, she said, "it was tedious and expensive and didn't help."

Despite being bedridden, she was still obliged to fulfill previously booked speaking engagements. Any traveling, even to the store, was an ordeal. "I needed a wheelchair in the airport and department stores. When I wasn't in a wheelchair, I walked with a cane," she remembered. It was on one particularly frustrating trip to the airport when she decided she'd had enough and wanted to regain her independence.

So she started to do the *Classical Stretch* workouts every day. "Soon after starting the workouts on a regular basis, I didn't have to swing my leg to move it; I could actually move my leg in a normal way," she said. "My life is so different now! I can walk normally. I have a high level of functioning. I think I would have just continued to experience a decrease in my strength and my ability to walk normally if I didn't do Essentrics."

In addition to dealing with debilitating physical pain, Sharon found herself battling prescription drug addiction. In her career, she had worked tirelessly as an advocate against substance abuse—even spending five years as the director of a clinical program for women detoxing from drugs. Sharon had a clear intellectual understanding of addiction, and knew all too well the familial, social, and psychological consequences of substance abuse. But she never thought she would find herself in the position of needing help herself. It was during an event she attended, in which one of the speakers related the story of a family member's battle with prescription pain medication, that Sharon realized she had a problem.

Summoning the mental determination to stop taking OxyContin and other painkillers wasn't hard for Sharon. However, dealing with the physical side effects of withdrawal was! "It was like being a junkie withdrawing from heroin," Sharon recalled. "I detoxed at home. And it was just terrible. I would get nausea in the evening. Itching and nausea and chills." But she suffered through the agony of detox and won.

Sharon is by no means alone. Tragically, dependency on pain medication has reached epidemic proportions in North America in tandem with the spread of chronic pain. Of the 9.4 million Americans who take opioids for long-term pain, 2.1 million are estimated by the National Institutes of Health to be addicted and are in danger of turning to the black market. Thankfully, Sharon was able to catch herself before that happened. More than a decade after discovering *Classical Stretch* on PBS, Sharon still practices it daily as a proactive approach to maintaining a pain-free body.

The following rebalancing workout should be done daily in its entirety to relieve and prevent back pain. (The first series of exercises is what finally helped me get rid of my chronic back pain!) If you are in pain, remain relaxed and never force your body to do anything that hurts. Try to do the workout feeling as comfortable and relaxed in your body as possible. Make sure to have a chair nearby for support.

If you feel a sharp pain while exercising, stop immediately, wait for the pain to subside, and restart slowly, inching forward so as not to retrigger the pain. The trick to long-term back pain relief is to do daily or twice-daily mini workouts in a pain-free mode.

Let me repeat that: Never work *through* the pain—always stop when you feel pain and restart after the pain has subsided.

ZOMBIE SWINGS

Zombie swings are designed to decompress the vertebrae as your spine hangs partially upside-down swinging in semi-traction. This helps pull the vertebrae apart, instantly relieving back pain and muscle tension. The stretching seems to unglue and liberate the large sheets of fascia that surround your back, preventing movement.

Do these swings as often as you like; they are great instant pain relievers. You may feel some pain as you first move; pause to let the pain dissipate, and then keep moving. The pain should go away within seconds.

Side view:

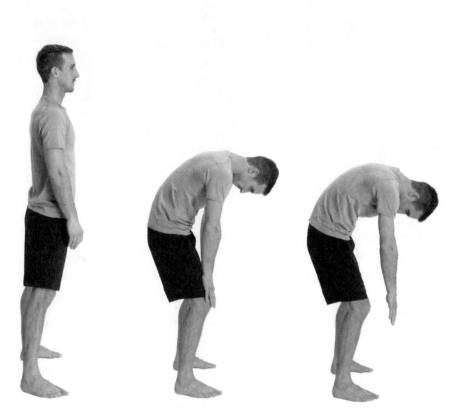

Front view:

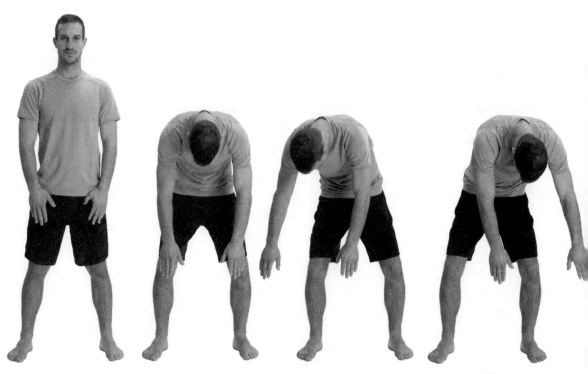

1. Stand with your feet parallel in a comfortably wide stance. Keep your muscles loose and relaxed.

2. Breathe deeply before beginning; this will help you focus on relaxing your muscles.

3. Tuck your tailbone under your hips (never stick your bum out), and bend your knees.

4. Slowly walk your fingertips down the fronts of your thighs; stop when you arrive at your knees.

5. Relax your neck as you lower your head forward.

6. Slowly sway side to side 4 to 8 times.

7. Slowly roll up one vertebra at a time to your starting position.

8. Repeat 2 more times.

9. Do this exercise as often as you want throughout the day.

OPEN-CHEST SWAN SEQUENCE

This sequence is designed to liberate your spine as you pull your torso upward. Combined with the zombie swings, it will rebalance your entire torso, relieving back, neck, and shoulder pain. It engages every muscle of the torso: the upper back, lower back, spine, pectorals, rectus abdominals, and latissimus dorsi. This feel-good sequence will rapidly release pain.

Front View:

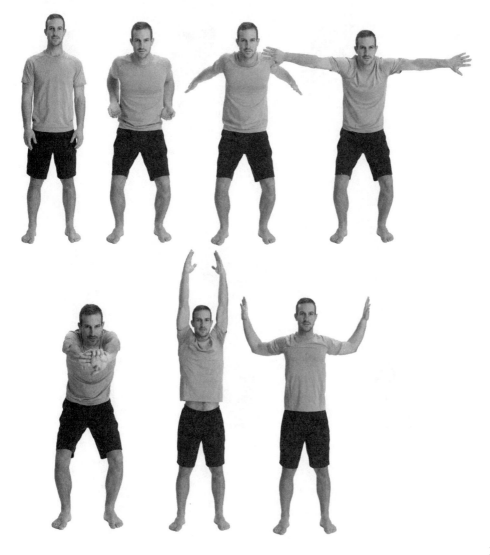

Side View:

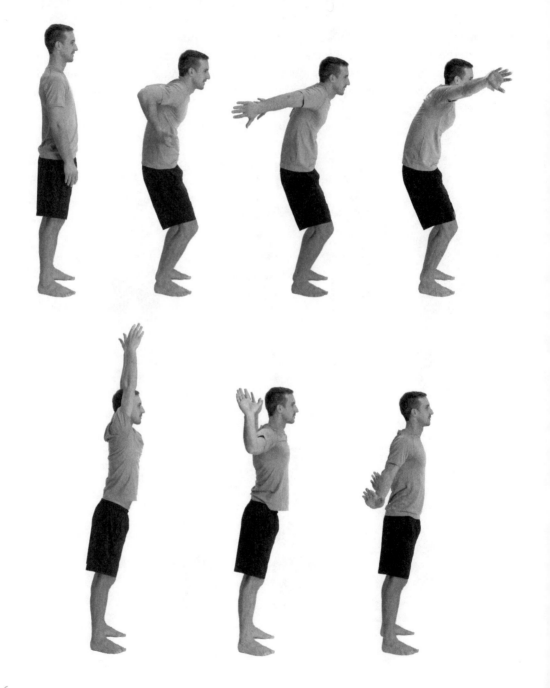

1. Stand with your feet shoulder-width apart.

2. Round your spine, tucking your tailbone under your hips while lifting and dropping your upper back forward and lifting your shoulders as high as possible.

3. Bend your knees and elbows, bringing your bent elbows beside your waist.

4. Draw your arms behind your back, straightening them; lift your shoulders as high as possible.

5. Slowly draw your arms from the back to the front until you can clasp your hands together.

6. Keep your arms in front of you with your hands held together, back rounded, and knees bent.

7. Shift your hips and ribs around, doing a kind of self-massage of your shoulders and spine.

8. Release your hands and slowly raise your arms above your head as you straighten your back and legs.

9. Angling your spine forward slightly, reach as high as you can toward the ceiling. Keep leaning slightly forward, and open your arms behind your shoulders while slightly bending the elbows.

10. Slowly straighten your elbows. Note: This exercise should feel like you are opening giant swan's wings. Your chest should be open to the ceiling while you keep your shoulders pressed down.

11. Repeat the full sequence 3 to 4 times.

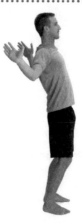

Incorrect Posture for Open-Chest Swan

A common mistake when doing this exercise is to lean backward, letting your weight sink into your lower spine (lumbar vertebrae) as you open your arms. This position is really bad for the spine, as it will compress and overload the vertebrae. Back pain often begins with compression of the spine. Always keep your spine and weight forward and pull upward with each vertebra to maintain a decompressed spine.

CEILING REACHES FOR BACK

This simple exercise will rebalance and decompress your spine by stretching and strengthening the back muscles. The rebalancing benefits come as you reach one arm at a time toward the ceiling. This enables you to stretch dozens of muscles along and around your spine that otherwise never get stretched to their maximum length.

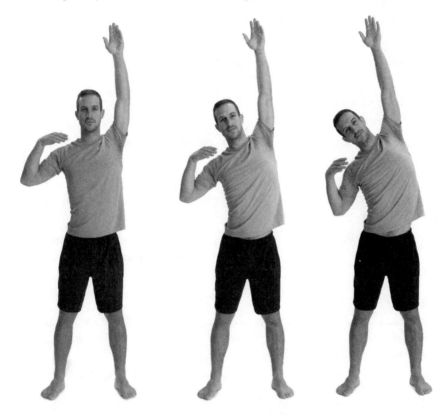

1. Start in an open stance with your feet slightly wider than your hips.
2. Raise one arm to the ceiling.
3. Relaxing the shoulders, count to 3 while trying to reach higher toward the ceiling.
4. Contract the shoulder muscles, gripping them as tightly as possible for the count of 3.

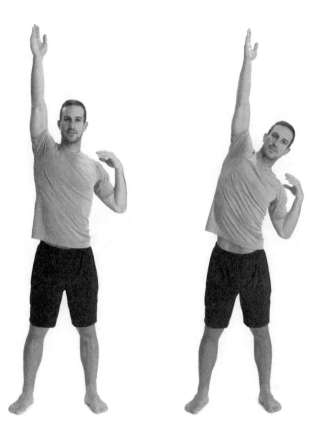

5. Relax them and, again, reach as high toward the ceiling as possible, letting the shoulder lift up as you reach.

6. Count to 3 while reaching higher.

7. Repeat the contract-relax-reach sequence 3 times before changing sides.

8. Repeat 4 times, alternating sides between each ceiling reach.

PUSH A PIANO/PULL A DONKEY SEQUENCE

I call this sequence "push a piano" and "pull a donkey," because these are two images that are easy for anyone to visualize and mimic. This sequence is aimed at relieving back pain by engaging all of your torso's muscles to rebalance: chest, abdominals, spine, lower back, shoulders, and side muscles. But this series also uses your hips, legs, knees, and feet, so it really is a full-body rebalancing sequence. This sequence also incorporates PNF (see box on page 135).

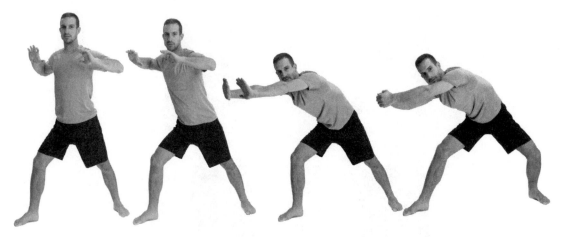

1. Stand in a comfortable front lunge, with your front leg bent and your back leg straight.

2. Your front and back knees should be correctly aligned over your feet. Imagine that you are pushing a piano; this image will make your back muscles contract. Note: You can adjust the image if you want to work less or more by simply imagining a light piano on rollers or a heavy grand piano.

3. Push the imaginary piano, taking 3 to 6 seconds from start to end of the push.

4. When you arrive at your maximum reach, relax your back muscles; when your back muscles relax, you'll be capable of bending forward a little farther.

5. Now imagine you are pulling a stubborn donkey; grab the rope and start pulling! Bend your back leg and tuck your tailbone under.

6. As you pull the imaginary donkey, your weight should shift from your front leg to your back leg.

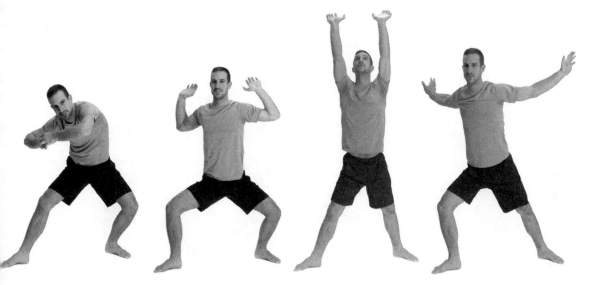

7. As you slowly pull the donkey toward you, your back muscles will contract.

8. Once you have pulled the donkey for 3 to 6 seconds, relax all your muscles. (It takes a few seconds to fully relax.) Move into a tai chi plié (see page 99), with both legs wide apart, feet turned out comfortably, knees bent, and back completely straight. Note: This is *not* a squat with your bum sticking out and your back leaning forward.

9. Imagine you are lifting heavy weights above your head; again, the image will make your muscles contract as you lift the heavy weight slowly above your head. When you have finished lifting the imaginary weights, relax your shoulders for about 3 seconds as you let the weights fly away.

10. Return to a front lunge and pull your arms behind you as you bend your body forward. Note: This is the same position as at the end of the open chest swan sequence on page 147.

11. Repeat this full sequence slowly 3 times per side before changing sides.

SIDE-TO-SIDE WINDOW WASHES FOR BACK

Your spine is designed to bend in many directions. When you have back pain, you don't want to bend your spine at all in fear of triggering more pain. Do these window washes in a relaxed manner, and you will slowly loosen the tight, painful muscles and get some relief. This exercise will increase the flexibility and strength of the muscles that support your spine when you do simple things all day long, such as get in and out of bed or the car, or as you put on a sweater or a pair of pants.

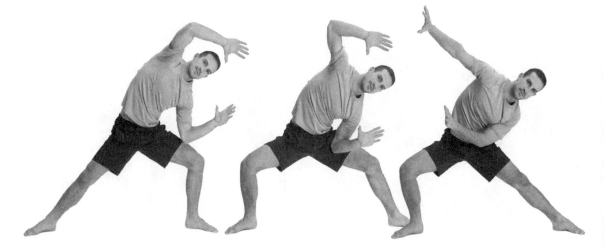

1. Start in a side lunge, bending sideways with your arms framing your head and your elbows bent.

2. Imagine you are standing close to a window while you are washing it. Open your fingers as wide as possible throughout the exercise.

3. Keep your elbows bent and your forearms beside your ears as you wash the window, sweeping your arms across your body.

4. Shift your ribs, feeling a stretch in them as you bend your torso while lunging side to side.

5. Throughout this sequence, imagine that you are pressed between two plates of glass, one in front of you and one behind; this image will help you keep your back straight and upright. When you have bent as far as you can, change sides; let your torso sway sideways as you change sides.

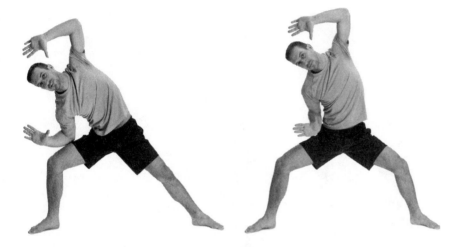

6. Alternate sides with each wash at least 8 times, and don't stop between each side—keep flowing from one side to the next.

> **Modification Note:**
> To make the exercise more strengthening: Imagine that you are washing a sticky substance off a window. This will make your muscles contract as you move.
> To make the exercise easier: Imagine that you are wiping the windows with a silk cloth. This will keep your muscles relaxed.

HIP SEQUENCE FOR BACK

When your hips are tight and immobile, the tension spirals into all the surrounding parts of your body, from your back into your legs. This hip sequence will loosen and stretch all of the many muscles that make up the hips, releasing any muscle chains that might be causing you back pain.

Be aware that the hips are attached to the spine and thighbone—which is why hip stretches simultaneously stretch the spine and hamstring muscles.

Phase One:

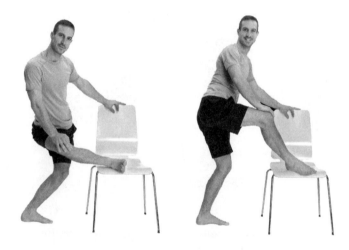

1. Stand beside your chair, placing your outside foot onto the seat while holding the back chair for balance.

2. Very slowly lower and raise your hip, keeping the knee of your standing leg bent.

3. You will feel a stretch in your hips as you raise and lower them.

4. The more you exaggerate the hip shifts, the better it will loosen the joint.

5. Repeat the raising and lowering of your hips at least 4 times, trying to dig deeper into the hip socket with each movement.

6. Repeat 4 times on each side.

Phase Two:

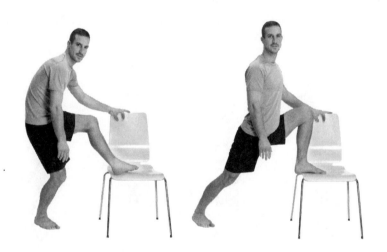

1. Face your chair and lift your outside knee straight to the ceiling.

2. Shift between rounding and straightening your back.

3. When you straighten your spine, shift the entire weight of your body forward toward the chair.

4. When you round the spine, shift your weight onto the back leg. As you shift from arch to straight, you will most likely find a tight spot. When you find a tight spot, slowly wiggle, trying to gently dislodge the blockage.

5. Repeat 4 times on each side.

PSOAS AND QUADRICEPS SEQUENCE FOR BACK

The psoas muscles are two long muscles that start at the front of the femur (thighbone) and thread through a space in the pelvic and hip bones, dividing into five muscles and attaching to the five lumbar vertebrae (lower spine). When the psoas muscle group is tight, it pulls on the lower spine, forcing the lower back to be in a permanently tucked-under position. A contracted psoas shortens the length of your stride; slows down your ability to walk, run, and climb stairs; makes it more difficult to comfortably get into or out of an easy chair (or on and off a toilet!); and generally interferes with ease of almost all movements.

A tight, unbalanced psoas is one of the major causes of chronic back pain. This exercise will stretch and rebalance the psoas, relieving back pain and giving you greater ease of movement.

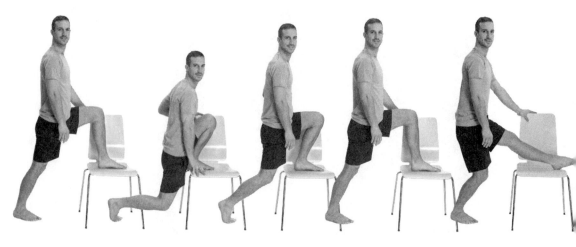

1. For the psoas stretch, face the seat of your chair; hold the back of the chair for balance. Note: Don't stand too close to the chair.

2. Place one foot flat on the seat of the chair.

3. Shift your body forward so that your weight is completely on the foot on the chair.

4. Do a pelvic tuck by tucking your tailbone under.

5. Raise your back heel.

6. Bend your back knee.

7. Tuck under your lower spine again.

8. Try to straighten your back leg while pressing your back heel into the floor and maintaining the pelvic tuck. You will probably feel a deep stretch at the front and top of your leg. That is correct!

9. Return to the starting position. Repeat this psoas stretch slowly 3 times on each leg.

10. For the quadriceps stretch, try to touch the floor with the knee of your standing leg.

11. The moment you arrive at your maximum depth, lift up and return to a straight leg.

12. Repeat the quadriceps stretch 3 times on each leg.

STANDING HAMSTRING STRETCH FOR BACK

Your hamstring muscles are located along the back of your leg. They are some of the longest muscles in your body. When they are tight, they will pull your lower back, forcing it to tuck under as they slowly unbalance your vertebrae. Maintaining flexibility in the hamstrings is extremely important for preventing and relieving back pain. Tight, unbalanced hamstrings are one of the major causes of back pain.

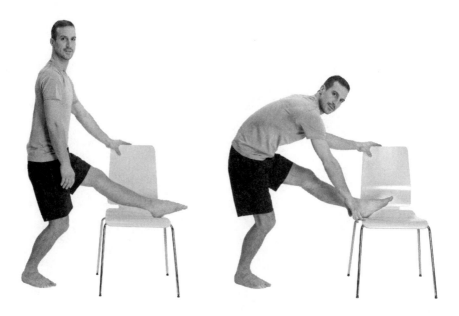

1. Stand beside your chair and place one leg on the chair. Try to straighten that knee. Note: Don't worry if you can't keep your knee bent—most people can't!

2. Holding the back of the chair for balance, bend your standing leg.

3. Slowly bend forward, trying to touch your foot; keep gently reaching over your foot for about 6 seconds.

4. Straighten your back and wiggle your body to relax all your muscles.

5. Repeat 4 times before changing legs.

HAMSTRING WINDMILL SEQUENCE FOR BACK

Tight hamstring muscles are often the cause of back pain because they pull the spinal muscles downward, compressing the spine. This sequence will stretch your hamstring muscles in addition to working your full spinal musculature.

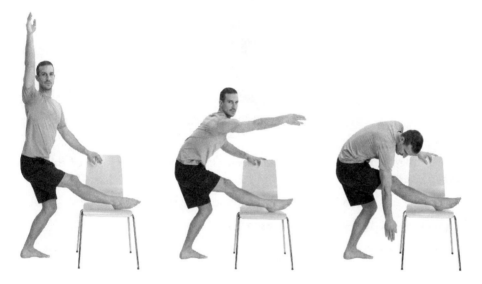

1. Stand beside your chair. Put your outside leg on the seat.

2. Holding the chair with one hand and keeping your standing knee slightly bent, lift the arm on the same side as your lifted leg above your head, while dropping the hip of the lifted leg down toward the ground.

3. Reach over your leg. You will feel a stretch in your hamstring.

4. Gently sweep your arm toward the floor. You will continue to feel a stretch in your hamstring.

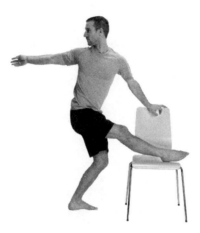

5. While straightening your back, twist your spine toward the back of the room and sweep your arm behind you.

6. Raise your arm above your head and continue into the next windmill.

7. Slowly repeat 3 to 4 windmills on each side.

• •

Incorrect Posture

When doing hamstring stretches, do not raise your hips. Bend the standing leg, relax the hip muscles, and push the hips down.

• •

CHAPTER 10

The Upper Back and Shoulder Workout

Carol Smith describes herself as having "an extreme personality," but unlike so many people who make that claim, she has the history to prove it.

In her forties, Carol decided to become a massage therapist and enrolled in a three-year college training program. She had never even had a massage. By the time she was in her sixties, Carol owned a massage clinic. It was then that she was introduced to the Essentrics program. After doing one workout, she knew she wanted to teach the method. Soon she made plans to travel thousands of miles to take a teacher-training course in Canada.

Most of the would-be teachers at the Essentrics workshop she attended had completed at least some online training or had previously attended one or two levels of instruction. Not Carol—she'd only leafed through the course outline before courageously signing up for all four levels of instruction. "I arrived knowing nothing about the program really. I was going to learn it all at once," she said. "That's me: Go big or go home."

Carol said that the day before she went through the training, she tried to buy some fitness clothes at a popular athletic store—but nothing fit her correctly, so she left empty-handed. Only one week later, Carol's entire body completely transformed—she returned to the same store and bought a whole new wardrobe of workout apparel. The clothes fit because her shape had changed dramatically.

As a toddler, Carol fell down some veranda stairs onto a broken bottle, cutting the nerves, tendons, and muscles of her left wrist. The childhood injury resulted in a lot of nerve damage and permanent paralysis to some finger muscles, leaving them incapable of straightening. To this day, Carol's hand remains in a permanent, semi-rounded ball shape. The semi-paralysis left her with an imbalance affecting the muscle chains in her left arm, starting at her fingers and going through her wrist, arm, shoulder, and spine into her upper back. Carol compensated for her weak left side by using her right hand and arm to do all the work. This led to major full-body muscular imbalances, with her right side overpowering the left. Her torso was visibly lopsided, with one shoulder positioned two inches above the other.

"I went on with my life, but over the years I had lost the rotation of my arm. Strangely, I never realized that my arm wasn't working correctly until I came to the Essentrics teacher training," she recalled. "All my life, I knew I never could get my shoulders straight—but figured if I worked harder at the gym I'd be able to get my shoulders back."

Little did Carol know that her problem was not simply getting her shoulders back but ungluing locked joints and reversing shrunken, atrophied muscles. She was compensating for the injured hand by locking her shoulder and arm joints and using her back muscles to do their work. "Looking back now, I see that all the experts who watched me for years, doing massages or fitness trainers, couldn't help straighten me out because they didn't know any better," she explained. "No one, not my college professors, not fitness trainers, ever mentioned locked joints, imbalanced muscles, or incorrect body movement." Her massage instructors looked at her hand as a handicap, not as an opportunity to find a solution.

When Carol became a masseuse, her lack of finger dexterity prevented her from doing a softer, more complex massage. And when the work required that she apply a lot of pressure with her left hand, Carol would put her right hand on top of her left to add to the pressure—but that approach was putting a lot of stress on both of her shoulders.

About ten years into her massage career, Carol developed excruciating pain in her right shoulder, in the area between the shoulder blades. She received regular massage therapy and chiropractic care, but between clients, she remembered, she'd find a corner of a wall to rub her shoulder blades against, trying to get rid of the pain.

At the same time the shoulder-blade pain started, she also began suffering severe migraine headaches. Once the migraines started coming more often, she took frequent sabbaticals, but there was no permanent escape from the physical work, as Carol regularly filled in for staff on their sick or vacation leaves. She was in agony.

Carol's daughter-in-law introduced her to *Aging Backwards* and the Essentrics program. The logic behind the program "resonated with me," she said. Within months of watching the program, she attended the teacher-training workshops.

Strange as it may seem in retrospect, prior to attending the workshops Carol hadn't realized that her back was lopsided. Most people normally favor one leg or the other. Carol was aware that she had poor posture, but she had no clue why. At the teacher training, I asked her to stand in front of the group and look at herself in the mirror—and she was shocked to see that one shoulder was two inches higher than the other. The mirror pointed out the severe structural imbalances in Carol's skeletal alignment and the immobility of her joints.

For the first time in her life, Carol understood that her alignment was seriously out of whack. The shocking part was that once she understood, it took her all of 20 minutes to make a physical change. Not only was Carol's alignment rapidly corrected, she was freed from decades of crippling shoulder pain.

"Miranda brought me to the front of the class and asked that I attempt to rotate my [left] arm in the joint. It was kind of glued. When I first tried to rotate my arm my whole body moved as one giant block," Carol recalled. "Very, very gently she showed me how to rotate my arm separately from the shoulder. Miranda was trying to get me to unlock my shoulder joint. Suddenly, it started to move separately from my shoulder. I wasn't up there more than ten minutes when I again looked at myself in the mirror and saw a new me. My shoulders had naturally adjusted themselves to become the same height and my spine had straightened. Best of all was that my stomach wasn't protruding! It was very emotional for me and everyone there!"

Not only did Carol's shoulders and back straighten out, her movements rapidly became more fluid. Decades of crippling shoulder pain vanished in minutes, as did the migraine headaches that she'd suffered for years: "There's no pain in my body anymore! In the past when I got a pain, I would think, 'Hmm, old age creeping up on me.' It is so exciting to know that it doesn't have to creep up on you."

Carol's childhood injury to her hand caused nerve damage that led to muscle imbalances that spiraled from her arm into her shoulder and back. With that type of injury, imbalances inevitably place stress on shoulder-blade musculature. The locked, immobilized shoulder joint caused a chain of damage to all her soft tissue, fasciae, and muscles. The immobility of her hand led to congealing of fasciae in her upper back as well as muscular atrophy of her shoulder, back, spine, and arm. The muscular imbalance forced one shoulder to be about two inches higher than the other, leading to permanent side flexion of the thoracic spine. The forward rotation of the left arm led to a permanent forward flexion of the spine. This led her lower spine to compensate the weight imbalance by forcing the pelvic spine to tuck under. It was the tucking under of the lower spine that made her stomach protrude—not carbs!

Simply rotating the arm within the shoulder socket loosened the congealed joint, returning mobility to the shoulder joint. As she rotated the arm within the joint all the other imbalances immediately corrected themselves. The primary technique used with Carol was rotation within a joint, but we also used the other principal techniques of the program to rebalance her muscles and realign her musculature.

Not everybody will get the instantaneous results that Carol did. Remember that Carol had already spent a week doing hours of daily Essentrics exercises in the workshops before she experienced that dramatic transformation. All 650 of her muscles had been stretched and strengthened, and all 384 of her joints had been rotated and loosened for hours each day. Her body was fully prepared for what seemed like a miraculously rapid adjustment. In reality, her body's change took place over hours of correct full-body exercise—exactly what is possible for you!

RIB SEQUENCE FOR UPPER BACK AND SHOULDERS

We have twelve pairs of ribs; all of which are attached to our spine at the back of our body and ten that are attached directly or indirectly to the sternum in front. The lower two pairs, called floating ribs, do not attach to the sternum. There are hundreds of short muscle fibers attaching the ribs to one another. These tiny muscles start at the front of each rib and continue the full length of each rib to the back. Every time we take a deep breath, these muscles expand like thick elastic bands permitting the rib cage as a whole to inflate like a giant balloon—and when we exhale, the ribs deflate. Every time we take a breath or move a muscle, the rib muscles expand and contract.

Intertwined and surrounding the ribs are complex structures of connective tissue. When the rib muscles atrophy from disuse, the connective tissue gets firmer, limiting the rib cage's range of motion. The ribs are intended to protect our heart, lungs, and stomach. Therefore, they must be capable of expanding, shrinking, twisting, turning, and bending. When the rib muscles become unbalanced, due to shrinkage or injury, we experience a tremendous amount of shoulder and upper-back pain. This sequence stretches and strengthens your valuable rib muscles.

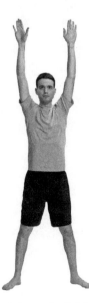

1. Stand with your feet slightly apart, legs straight. Raise your arms above your head.

2. Slowly inhale and exhale several times, consciously trying to expand your rib cage. Each breath should last about 6 to 10 seconds. After several slow, deep breaths, your spinal muscles will have loosened and you might be capable of reaching your arms considerably higher than before.

3. Slowly bend sideways until you feel the ribs stretching.

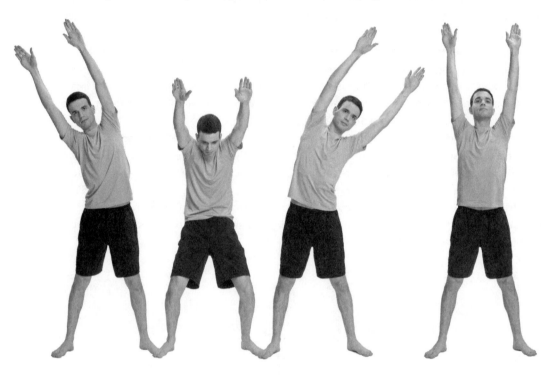

4. Straighten and then start to draw an imaginary small circle on the ceiling with your fingers. The objective of this exercises is to stretch the front, side, back, and front rib muscles as you follow the circle.

5. Reach as far as you can above your head, keeping your elbows as straight as possible. The arm muscles are connected to the ribs through muscle chains; you're using them to fully stretch and strengthen your ribs.

6. As you follow the circle on the ceiling, slowly rotate to the back, side, front, and side again.

7. Keep your legs and back straight when you rotate to the side and back. However, when you rotate to the front, bend your knees and round your spine.

8. Repeat the rib rotations, very slowly, 2 to 3 times in each direction.

• •

Incorrect Spine Posture

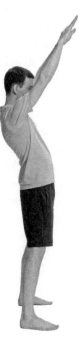

We have a tendency to sink into our lower spine when standing upright. This is the most common incorrect spine posture. Over time, the muscles of our spine and torso slowly will reshape themselves, adjusting to the imbalance by shrinking and atrophying, leading to imbalance and back pain. When the lower spine is sunken, the upper spine must droop forward to compensate for the incorrect distribution of body weight.

Look at yourself sideways, in a mirror, to check your posture. If you are sinking into your lower spine, it usually takes several weeks (and sometimes months) of stretching and strengthening to rebalance the muscles. When you start making a change in your posture, the correct posture will feel *incorrect!* The weak, shrunken muscles won't be able to comfortably hold you upright, and the tight muscles will pull you backward into your old posture.

Be patient and know that the health, energy, pain relief, and beauty benefits of proper posture are well worth the effort!

• •

FROZEN SHOULDER BENT-ELBOW
FIGURE 8

Strong, flexible shoulder muscles depend on lots of arm movement. We should get plenty of arm and shoulder movement daily by doing ordinary chores: getting dressed, reaching into high cupboards, painting a room, carrying groceries, cooking, and doing laundry. But thanks to our labor-saving modern appliances, we hardly have to lift our arms in our daily activities anymore. This lack of arm use can lead to a condition called adhesive capsulitis (frozen shoulder). Shoulder, arm, wrist, or elbow accidents that require the arm to be immobilized in a sling can also lead to frozen shoulder. Many women suffer frozen shoulder after breast cancer surgery.

Frozen shoulder is excruciatingly painful. This is one time when you will need to move through the pain. Keep in mind that after a couple of days of gentle movement, your muscles will strengthen and the pain will dissipate. Take your time and stay relaxed through this entire sequence. The moment your shoulder muscles tighten or you feel any pain, stop moving and relax; let the pain subside before you continue. As I said in the previous paragraph, the pain may not totally subside when you first start these exercises.

If you have chronic pain, it may take extra minutes to complete this sequence. The secret to pain relief is to keep your body loose and limp. Never force your muscles—that will only cause further injury!

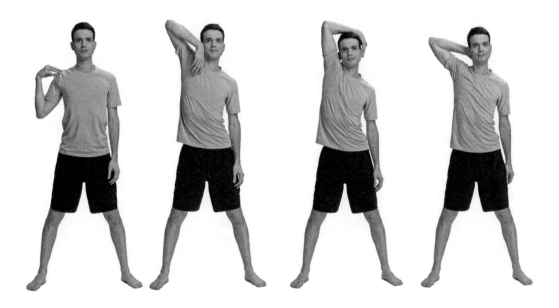

1. Stand with your feet apart, wider than your hips.

2. Raise your arm sideways and try to touch your shoulder with the fingers of that hand, leaving the other arm relaxed at your side.

3. Raise the elbow of your bent arm, while still trying to touch your shoulder.

4. As you lift your elbow above your head, let your forearm and hand rest gently on top of your head. Note: Keep your spine upright all the time. Do not bend sideways or use your torso in any way; move your arm independently from your shoulder joint.

5. Slowly move to try to touch the back of your neck.

6. Keep moving, pulling your arm to shoulder height.

7. Then return to the beginning position and repeat 4 times in a row on both sides.

8. Do this as often as you want during the day. (It may take a week or two of daily practice to get rid of frozen shoulder.)

FROZEN SHOULDER STRAIGHT-ARM FIGURE 8

This exercise is designed to be paired with the frozen shoulder bent-arm sequence (above). There are many shoulder muscles that can be engaged and stretched only when your arm is straight. This straight-arm exercise captures the muscles that the bent-arm sequence doesn't use. By pairing the two, we rebalance all the muscles of the upper body and shoulders. This sweeping figure 8 exercise is a full-body sequence that works muscles from the fingertips to the toes.

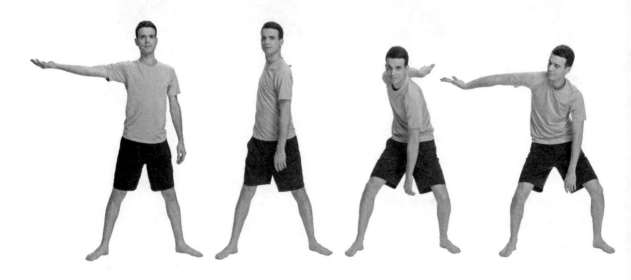

1. Standing with your feet comfortably wide apart, extend one arm to shoulder height, keeping the other relaxed at your side.

2. Rotate your spine toward the back of the room, turning in the direction of the extended arm. Bend your knees slightly, tuck your pelvis under, and round your back and upper body.

3. Gently rotate your back arm, twisting it within your shoulder socket.

4. Return to face the front while maintaining a maximum rotation of the arm within the shoulder socket.

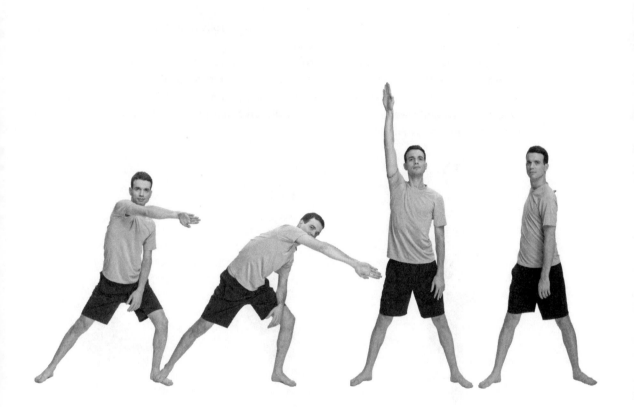

5. Gently sweep your rotated arm across the front of your body, keeping it rotated in your shoulder socket the entire time. Note: You may feel a pull through the entire musculature of your spine, from your shoulder through to your tailbone.

6. Shift your weight into a deep side lunge while sweeping the same arm toward the opposite wall.

7. Straighten your legs while lifting your arm above your head.

8. Finish the sequence by rotating the spine backward while lowering the arm to shoulder height behind you.

9. Repeat 3 to 4 times in a row on one side; then switch sides and repeat 3 to 4 times on the other side.

SPINE FLEXIBILITY SEQUENCE

Tight shoulders are often caused when the muscles of the spine become unbalanced: too weak, too strong, and/or too tight. This sequence will unlock the muscles of your spine, liberating compressed, damaged joints. While following these exercises, focus on the full spine and try to use every vertebra.

If some parts of your spine won't move, which is very common, don't give up. Keep trying to move them even if they don't budge—as long as you are not in pain. Do not focus on being perfect; rather, focus on feeling any movement in your spine. Even the tiniest movement means that you are slowly unlocking your joints and muscles. Over time, they will loosen up.

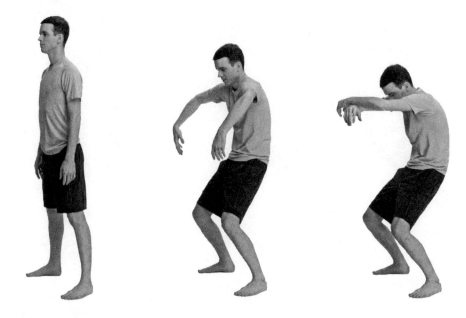

1. Stand straight with your feet apart and arms down.

2. Bend your knees, tuck your tailbone under, round your back, and raise your shoulders.

3. Lift your arms in front to shoulder height, keeping them relaxed.

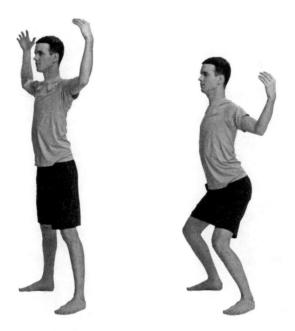

4. Raise your shoulders as high as possible.

5. Reverse the position by standing straight and lifting your arms over your head as you open your chest.

6. Pull your arms behind you, keeping your elbows bent, lowering your shoulders. Imagine that you are slipping your shoulder blades into your back pockets.

7. At the same time, bend your knees and arch your back by sticking out your bum.

8. Return to starting position.

9. Repeat this sequence slowly at least 8 times in a row.

ARM CIRCLES

These shoulder-elongating arm circles use all the muscles required to lift and lower your arms and shoulders. They will help you regain and maintain excellent range of motion of the arms and shoulders.

When arm and shoulder muscles are unbalanced, weak, or tight, our arms become difficult to lift, causing us to suffer from neck and back pain.

This exercise is also designed to open your chest, strengthen your upper-back muscles, and improve your posture.

NOTE: This exercise is much more difficult than it looks! Don't be shy to stop anytime you'd like, shake out your arms, and resume when you're ready.

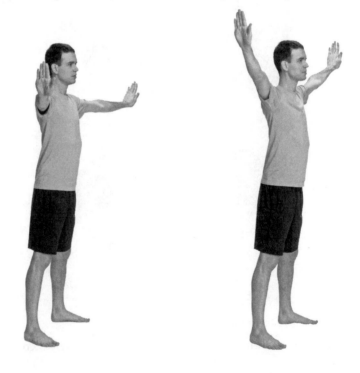

1. Stand in a wide stance and raise your arms sideways to shoulder height, hands flexed at the wrists.

2. Keep the shoulders down and imagine you are pulling your arms out of your shoulder sockets.

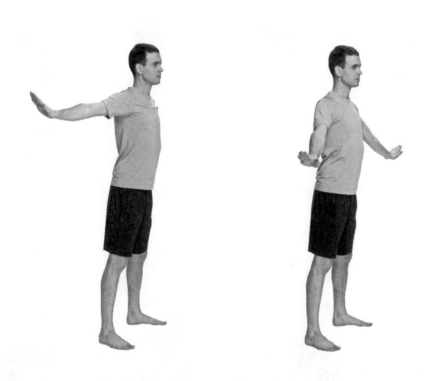

3. With your arms extended straight out to the sides at shoulder height, draw 8 small circles, moving only your arms. Hold your shoulders down to make sure they don't move.

4. Reverse the direction and draw 8 circles in the opposite direction.

STAR ARM SEQUENCE

This sequence will stretch, strengthen, and rebalance your shoulders and upper back.

Side View:

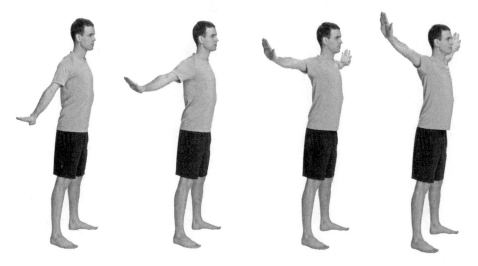

Front View:

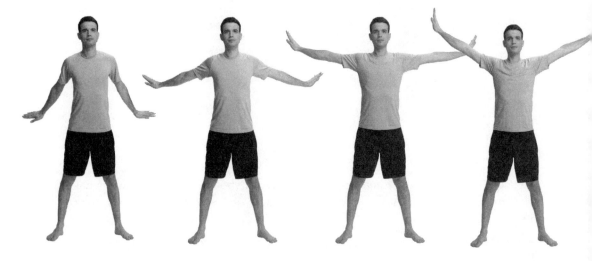

1. Stand in a comfortably wide stance. Aim to keep your spine straight, maintaining perfect posture with your weight forward and your shoulders down throughout the exercise.

2. Lift your arms to shoulder height, flex your wrists, and extend your arms outward, imagining that you are trying to pull your arms out of the shoulder joints. Note: Your shoulders will naturally want to lift every time you lift your arms. It's important to keep your shoulders down to lengthen the shoulder muscles, which is essential for decompressing your neck and back.

3. Pump your arms slowly, as far behind you as possible, without moving your back. Aim for points near your hips, below your shoulders, above your shoulders, and above your head. (Imagine that you are touching different points of a star.)

4. Don't jerk or force your arms as you pump them backward.

5. Do 4 pumps up and 4 pumps down to make one star.

6. Repeat the star 8 times.

SPINE STRETCH SEQUENCE USING A CHAIR

This stretch works as a self-massage for the full spine and hips. Take your time here and indulge in any part of this sequence that feels good. When you hold on to the back of the chair, it allows you to relax into the stretch without worrying about losing your balance and without contracting your spinal muscles.

NOTE: Always protect your joints when exercising. In this sequence, do not allow your body strength or weight to overwhelm the shoulder joints by forcing them into a deeper stretch than they are capable of.

Phase One:

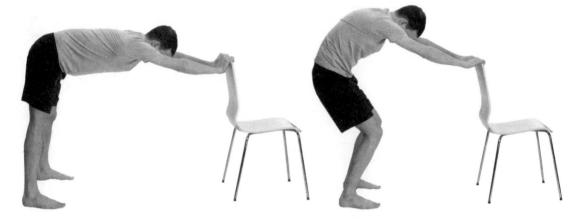

1. Start by facing your chair. Place your feet apart and hold the back of the chair with both hands.

2. Bend your knees and try to straighten your spine into a tabletop position.

3. Stand far enough away from the chair to be able to form a tabletop flatness of your back. Relax into this position, taking about 3 to 5 seconds Note: Many people are incapable of flattening their back. Do your best without forcing your spine to be straight.

4. Then step a little closer to the chair, slightly straighten your knees, and round your spine in a catlike arch. Walk your feet backward, returning to the starting tabletop position.

5. Repeat 4 to 8 times, alternating from rounded to straightened spine and back again.

Phase Two:

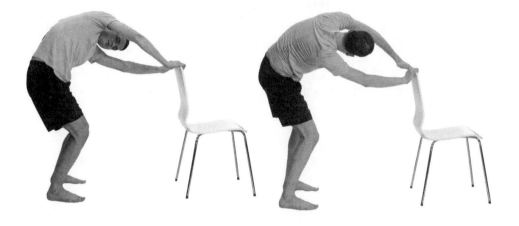

1. With your hands fixed on the back of your chair and your spine slightly rounded, shift your weight onto one leg, bending that knee.

2. Rotate your torso toward the bent knee until you feel a stretch in your shoulders, back, and hips.

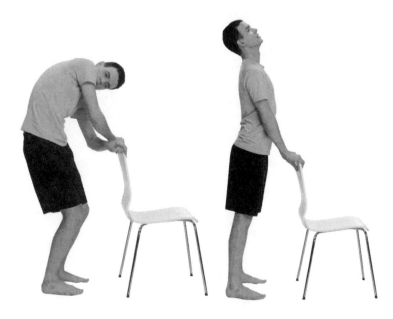

3. Take 8 to 10 seconds per leg, and alternate 4 times each direction.

4. Walk closer to the chair, straightening your knees slightly.

5. Once you are close to the chair, repeat the rotation in step 2. (It will stretch different muscles of your spine than the lower position.)

6. Take 8 to 10 seconds per leg, and alternate 4 times each direction.

7. Stand completely straight, holding the chair, and lift your head to pull your neck and face toward the ceiling.

CHAPTER 11

The Connective Tissue Workout

Sara Landau is an internationally renowned and sought-after artist. She has also been, for many years, a sufferer of chronic pain. Throughout her life, Sara has had to contend with significant health obstacles. She was born with childhood epilepsy. The seizures began at birth and ended when she was nine. Both of her two most memorable seizures involved her elbow: it became caught in a door when she was six, and it was hit by a competitor's tennis racket when she was nine.

Epilepsy is a neurological condition that affects the nervous system. Seizures seen in epilepsy are caused by disturbances in the electrical activity of the brain. In most cases, people grow out of childhood epilepsy before adulthood, as did Sara.

Epilepsy didn't stop Sara from taking up ballet early in life. At eight, she joined a professional ballet school. At fifteen, she had to make a decision between a career in ballet or academics. She chose academics, which meant leaving the ballet school and joining a regular school, where she chose running as her physical activity. The strong, flexible muscles she had developed in her ballet training made her a star runner.

In those two years of high school, she did almost no preparatory physical training and still won every race. Then she went off to college, where she resumed taking daily ballet classes.

When she was regularly attending ballet classes, she never experienced knee pain.

However, during her six-week summer holidays, when she stopped dancing, she always suffered from knifelike knee pain. When she resumed her ballet classes, the pain would disappear and she'd be fine.

After college, she began her career as a painter. Her companion was a large friendly dog who required lots of daily walks. She'd sit for hours cross-legged, with a canvas leaning against the wall in front of her, and her palette and other tools spread out on either side. She'd reach, twist, turn, and bend all day as she went from palette to canvas. From ages twenty-two to twenty-nine, this is how she spent most of her waking hours—painting cross-legged.

During this period, Sara's knees were generally pain-free. Then she started to feel knee pain when she ran for a bus, played tennis, or moved quickly, which included walking her rambunctious dog. She stopped all running and sports, believing that she had bad knees. Still, it was impossible to stop her dog from pulling as they walked—which was when she began experiencing back pain. By age twenty-eight her back pain became impossible to ignore: she experienced numbness in one foot and acute back spasms, immobilizing her in bed. An MRI showed a minor bulging L4-L5 disc.

By then both her knee and back pain had progressed to a level of 5 on a scale of 1 to 10. "I just coped with all the different things that came my way, the bad knees, the bad back," Sara recalled. "I had physiotherapy. I went to see if I needed surgery, but it was never bad enough to need that. They suggested that I wear knee braces, which were cumbersome, so I didn't wear them. I really became inactive because things just hurt. I never ran. I would mostly walk or swim because everything else bothered my knees or my back."

At age thirty-one, her life changed with a diagnosis of Graves' disease, an autoimmune disease characterized by the overproduction of thyroid hormones (hyperthyroidism). The recommended treatment, which Sara underwent, was to completely destroy the thyroid gland through radiation and replace the thyroid function with daily medication.

Then in 2011, when she was thirty-seven, Sara's life changed once again, professionally and personally. She gave birth to twins—a healthy girl and boy—and unveiled her most famous work to date, a painting titled *Twin Children*.

Sara's pregnancy did not run smoothly; it had been extremely difficult. She was on strict bed rest for her early pregnancy. After five months, she was allowed to walk, but her muscles had atrophied to the point where she could barely stand. And just as she was regaining enough muscle mass to begin walking again, she experienced early labor contractions, common in women carrying twins. To prevent premature delivery, her doctor again ordered Sara to stay in bed throughout the remainder of her pregnancy.

By the time she was ready to deliver, her muscles had shrunk from extreme atrophy and were completely devoid of the strength required for a natural delivery. She gave birth by Cesarean section, which made recovery slow and painful. The combination of nine months in bed and a cesarean birth left her weak and in chronic pain. "I was almost completely atrophied," Sara recalled. "I had stayed in bed for almost a year. At first I could barely stand up. I could barely walk a block. When I eventually went to a grocery store, just to walk down one aisle left me completely out of breath. I had lost so much muscle mass that I had no strength. I had to have help to bathe the babies. Even assuming a bending position was extremely hard."

A physiotherapist who regularly treated Sara during her bed rest suggested that she try Essentrics after she delivered the babies, as a way to regain her strength. As soon as she could, Sara paid a visit to a studio where our classes are offered. "I loved it," Sara said. "The classroom setting was a familiar environment. Also, some of the stretching was similar to the movements suggested by my physiotherapist to maintain my back. So there was crossover."

However, with two babies to care for, there was no time left to care for herself and take regular classes. "I loved the classes, but there was no way I could go on a regular basis. I was breast-feeding and I didn't have the time or the strength." She dropped out of the classes, as motherhood was all she could handle. Sara, however, is nothing if not stoic: "I think we are all given what we can handle and we just have got to get through it. When you have two small babies, you don't have time to think about your pain. You only think about what is next to be done."

Then an accident forced her to focus on her own health. Her children were about two when Sara took them on their first airplane trip. "They were so excited that they ran to find their seats. As I ran after them I hit my knee on one of the seats. I felt a sharp pain and heard a loud pop." She sought medical attention at her destination, and an MRI when she got home showed that she had torn her meniscus (a band of cartilage within the knee joint).

Sara's doctors recommended that she bicycle to strengthen her knee. She was desperate to regain strength, but rather than bicycling she started doing *Classical Stretch* DVDs and eventually returned to our classes. Soon she was back exercising on a daily basis, and experiencing significant relief from both the knee and back pain. Still, her doctors recommended surgery to repair her torn meniscus. She considered it but ultimately decided to keep with her exercise program a little longer and see if she could avoid such an invasive procedure.

A year after rejecting the operation, Sara said the program not only helped her naturally repair her knee injury but also dramatically lessened her chronic knee and lower-back pain. Two years after starting the classes, she was close to being pain-free. Not only was she physically stronger as a result of Essentrics, but she had finally assumed control of her physical health.

"Essentrics has really helped," she said. "It has helped my back pain tremendously. I am definitely much stronger, although my knees are still a problem, but nothing like what they were. I do almost all the movements, but I don't do deep lunges or a deep plié. I wear knee braces to all the classes because I don't want to injure myself further. When I start to feel pain, I stop at that point."

What's interesting to me is that during her tenure as a ballet student, Sara had neither knee nor back pain. Her knee pain started and became acute when she was on vacation, not when she was exercising. As a ballet dancer, she could easily do the splits and had great flexibility. She complained of having difficulty in holding her legs in the high positions because her leg muscles were too weak. As a former ballerina, I know that holding your legs above hip height is difficult, so that was not relevant. But Sara's pain was affecting her whole life.

Sara's core issue was that she was constantly suffering from muscle atrophy. Her pain was all joint related: in her knees, elbow, and L4-L5 vertebra. The meniscus tear and other ligament tears were all in the joint.

It's important to look at Sara's muscles to understand why atrophy was causing her joint pain. Think of a muscle like a giant rubber band and the tendons as two ridged ropes attaching the muscle to the bones, making a joint. If the giant rubber band shrinks, it will pull on the ridged ropes. If the shrinking is sufficient, it will cause a dangerous pulling on the attachment points, squeezing the joints together. This is one reason why atrophy is extremely painful. Muscle atrophy becomes more common as we age, and without proper exercise it can become a serious issue (usually after age fifty).

It is rare for an active young person to suffer from atrophy unless the atrophy is triggered by a neurological disorder—which is, I believe, what happened in Sara's case. When she went back to ballet classes, where she stretched and strengthened her muscles, the pain disappeared. The times in her life when she did not regularly stretch and strengthen, she was in acute pain. Her college vacations and her bed rest during pregnancy led to her greatest pain. Everybody's muscles shrink when they stop doing regular exercise, but the normal rate of change is over years—not days, as in Sara's case.

The human body is mysterious. I believe that Sara's knee and back pain were triggered by a malfunctioning neurological message that caused her muscles to prematurely atrophy. She has a family history of neurological conditions, and she herself suffered twice from neurological disorders: childhood epilepsy and an autoimmune disorder of hyperthyroidism. Her conditions led to premature muscle and connective tissue atrophy. Many people who suffer from combinations of neurological disorders can use Essentrics to help relieve the symptoms.

When you are exercising to relieve pain related to connective tissue, it's important to move very slowly, giving the many paper-thin layers time to warm up and regain their essential sliding ability. Remember: When we don't use all of our muscles, the connective tissues surrounding them don't move either. As a muscle atrophies, the connective tissue around it congeals and hardens. The slow movements in this workout safely return the sliding action back to the connective tissue layers as the atrophied muscle regains its shape, strength, and flexibility. Make sure to have a chair nearby for support.

SPINAL ROLL AND OPEN-CHEST SWAN SEQUENCE

This exercise is a complete rebalancing sequence. The spinal roll will gently stretch and loosen the massive sheets of connective tissue in your back. As you gently roll down and up your vertebrae, you will feel a pulling sensation—that's your fascia being stretched. The slower you go, the better your chance of releasing much-needed fluids into the fascia. Those fluids will lubricate the thin sheets of fascia, making movement smooth and easy. When you move rapidly, the lubricating effects don't have time to work.

The open-chest swan exercise will loosen the tight connective tissue right down the front of your body; you will experience an amazing feeling of liberation, starting in your neck and going into your chest and abdomen.

Front View:

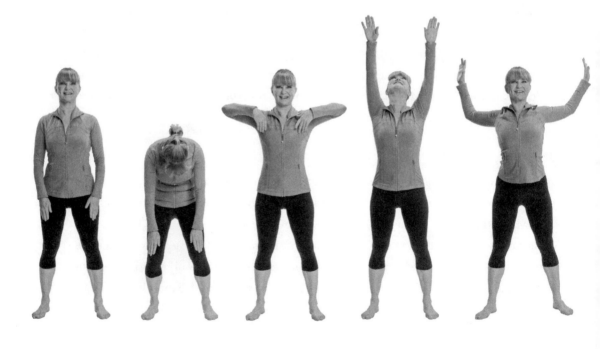

Side View:

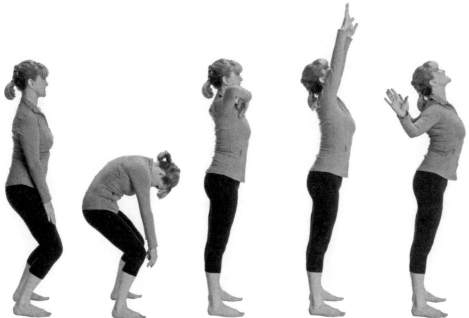

1. Place your feet hip-width apart and bend your knees. Tuck your tailbone under and keep your spine rounded; don't let your bum stick out.

2. Slowly walk your fingers down the front of your legs until you can touch your knees.

3. Permit your head to hang forward by relaxing your neck muscles.

4. Slowly sway from side to side when you are at the bottom of the spinal roll; as you sway, you should feel the sheets of connective tissue in your back being stretched and loosened. Don't rush through this, as it takes time for these tissues to restart sliding over each other after years of being glued together!

5. Slowly roll your spine up, one vertebra at a time, keeping your spine rounded and your tailbone tucked under. Keep your arms relaxed, hanging beside your body. As you roll up, let your fingers touch your body until you have fully straightened your spine.

6. Then, continuing your fingertips' motion, reach your arms above your head, trying to touch the ceiling. Try not to grip the shoulder muscles, because they will block your ability to reach higher.

7. To move into open-chest swan, open your chest as wide as you can. Bend your elbows while you pull your arms behind you. Note: Make sure you do not bend back or drop your weight in the lower spine. Keep your spine angled forward, even when pulling your arms behind you. Your arms should feel like large swan's wings in flight!

8. While doing this, imagine that you are slipping your shoulder blades into your back pockets.

9. Repeat the full spinal roll and open-chest swan sequence 3 times.

RIB SEQUENCE FOR CONNECTIVE TISSUE

Our ribs are intended to protect our heart, lungs, and stomach. Therefore, they must be capable of expanding and shrinking, twisting, turning, and bending as we go through our normal daily activities. When our rib muscles become unbalanced, due to shrinkage or injury, we can experience a tremendous amount of shoulder and upper-back pain. These exercises stretch and strengthen your valuable rib muscles.

SAFETY RULE

When bending forward, in almost every exercise, round your spine and tuck your tailbone under, unless otherwise directed.

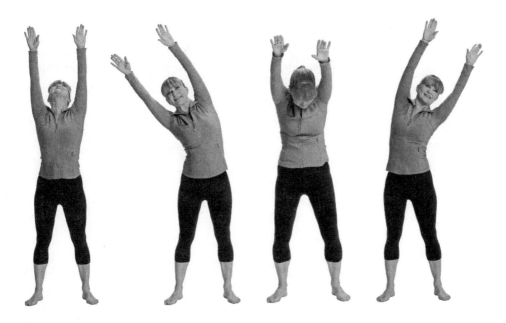

1. Stand with your feet slightly apart, legs straight. Raise your arms above your head.

2. Slowly inhale and exhale several times, consciously trying to expand your rib cage. Each breath should last about 6 to 10 seconds. (After several slow, deep breaths, your

spinal muscles will have loosened and you might be capable of reaching considerably higher than before.)

3. Slowly bend sideways until you feel the ribs stretching.

4. Start to draw a small imaginary circle with your fingers on the ceiling. (The objective of this exercise is to stretch the front, side, back, and front ribs as you follow the circle.)

5. Reach as far as you can above your head, keeping the elbows as straight as possible.

6. As you follow the circle on the ceiling, slowly rotate to the back, side, front, and side again.

7. Keep your legs and back straight when you rotate to the side and back; however, when you rotate to the front, bend your knees and round your spine.

8. Repeat the rib rotations, very slowly, 2 to 3 times in each direction.

Incorrect Posture

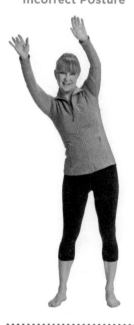

When bending sideways, do not lift your hip to follow the movement. Raising your hip will prevent any stretch from taking place. Hold your hip parallel to the floor when you are stretching sideways.

Correct Posture in Rib Sequence

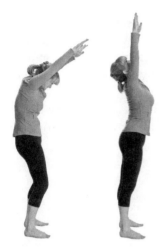

When your body tilts forward, your knees bend and your tailbone tucks under.

During the back rotation (ceiling reach), your spine should be pulling upward. Be aware not to sink the weight of your body into your lumbar vertebrae or lower spine.

Incorrect Posture in Rib Sequence

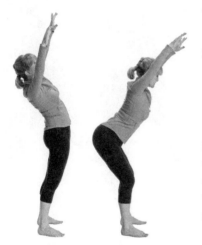

1. Do not sink your body weight into your lower spine, ever.

2. If you are incapable of raising your arms high enough to be in line with your ears while keeping perfect posture, stop at the level where you are comfortably capable of lifting them.

Do not stick out your bum when bending forward—doing so will put a lot of stress on your lower back and lumbar vertebrae. Sticking out your bum will also block your ribs from benefiting from the stretch.

WINDMILL SEQUENCE

The torso is intertwined and surrounded by massive sheets of connective tissue. All large full-body movements are very effective in gaining and maintaining healthy connective tissue. The windmill sequence is intended to elongate one side of the torso at a time. It gently stretches the large and small sheets of connective tissue that both restrict movement and cause pain.

Before beginning the actual windmill sequence, practice shifting your weight from one lunge to the other. This will familiarize you with the leg movement, making the full sequence easier to do when you add the arms.

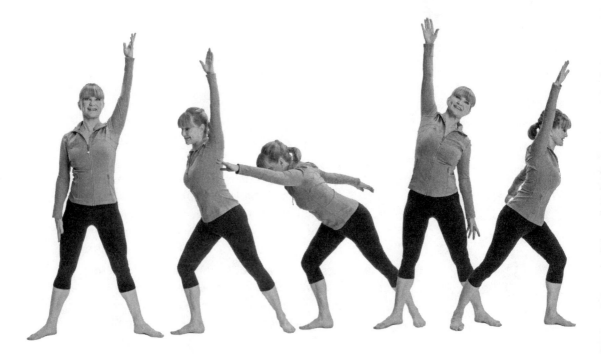

1. Stand in a comfortably wide stance, with your feet turned out and one arm raised above your head.

2. Turn your body to face a diagonal with the legs in a lunge, front knee bent and back leg straight with the heel flat on the floor.

3. Lower into a front lunge, pulling your arm diagonally forward. Note: You will notice that one side of your spine will be pulled more than the other side. Ensure that your

spine is always elongated as you bend forward. Be careful not to sink your weight into the lower spine.

4. Once you have shifted your weight into the lunge, start stretching the top arm toward the upper corner of the room and the bottom arm toward the lower back corner.

5. Begin to rotate your arms simultaneously in large circles, moving them like the blades of a windmill, while you remain in your lunge.

6. To change sides, return to the starting position using the opposite arm, pulling it as high as possible toward the ceiling.

7. Either repeat 4 very slow windmills per side or alternate 8 to 16 windmills, changing legs with each windmill.

SPINE STRETCH SEQUENCE USING A CHAIR

This stretch works to self-massage the full spine and hips. Take your time here and indulge in any part of this sequence that feels good. Holding on to the back of your chair allows you to relax into the stretch without worrying about losing your balance and without contracting the spinal muscles.

NOTE: Always protect your joints when exercising. In this exercise, do not allow your body strength or weight to overwhelm the shoulder joints by forcing them into a deeper stretch than your joints are capable of supporting.

Phase One:

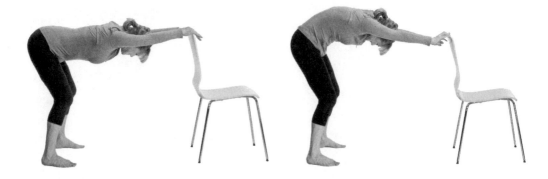

1. Start by facing your chair,

2. Stand far enough away from the chair in order to best straighten your spine with your feet apart while holding the back of the chair with both hands.

3. Bend your knees as you try to straighten your spine into a tabletop position.

4. After relaxing into this tabletop position for between 3 to 5 seconds, step a bit closer to the chair, while slightly straightening your knees, and rounding your spine in a catlike arch.

5. Gently move around in the catlike arch for 3 to 5 seconds.

6. Then walk your feet backward, returning to the starting tabletop position.

7. Repeat 4 to 8 times, alternating from rounded to straightened spine and back again.

Phase Two:

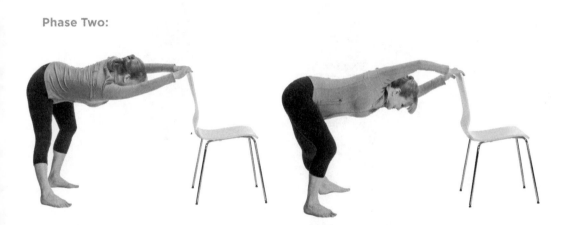

1. With your hands fixed on the back of your chair and your spine slightly rounded, shift your weight onto one leg, bending that knee.

2. Rotate your torso toward the bent knee until you feel a stretch in your shoulders, back, and hips.

3. Take 8 to 10 seconds per leg, and alternate 4 times each direction.

4. Walk closer to the chair, straightening the knees slightly.

5. Once you are close to the chair, repeat the rotation in step 2. (It will stretch different muscles of your spine than the lower position.)

6. Take 8 to 10 seconds per leg, and alternate 4 times in each direction.

7. Stand up straight, holding the chair and lifting your head to pull your neck and face toward the ceiling.

SPINE ROTATIONAL STRETCH

To be free of pain related to our connective tissue, we must move every muscle in the body, as connective tissue surrounds and intertwines every muscle. This exercise deeply increases the rotational mobility of the spine and full torso, using a deep muscle chain from the fingers through to the toes.

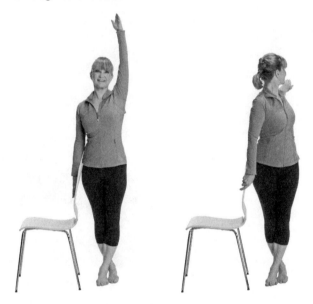

1. Stand with your right hip touching the back of your chair and your left foot crossed in front of your right foot.

2. Holding the chair, raise your other arm above your head, trying to touch the ceiling.

3. Slowly twist your spine away from the chair, rotating on your spine until you have twisted as far as possible.

4. As you rotate your torso, lower your arm, turn your head to follow your hand with your eyes. Finish by looking at the back of the room and at your back arm.

5. When you finish your spinal rotation, your arm should be shoulder height, with your fingertips reaching toward the back of the room.

6. Holding your arm at shoulder height, inhale deeply. Then exhale, trying to simultaneously reach farther toward the back of the room and rotate your spine a little farther.

7. Repeat slowly at least 4 times on each side.

FASCIA STRETCH FOR CONNECTIVE TISSUE

One of our largest sheets of fascia surrounds our thighs and hips; it's been referred to as our "tight shorts." These sheets of fascia can get twisted, making movement very painful. This hip sequence will loosen and stretch the fascia, helping it return to its natural shape and rapidly relieving fascial pain.

Phase One:

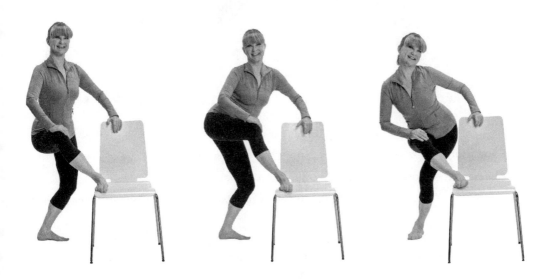

1. Stand beside your chair, placing your outside foot onto the seat while holding the back chair for balance.
2. Slowly lower and raise your hip, keeping the knee of your standing leg bent.
3. You will feel a stretch in the hips as you raise and lower your hips. The more you exaggerate the hip shifts, the better it will loosen the joint.
4. Repeat the raising and lower of your hips a least 4 times, trying to dig deeper into the hip socket with each movement.
5. Switch sides and repeat 4 times.

Phase Two:

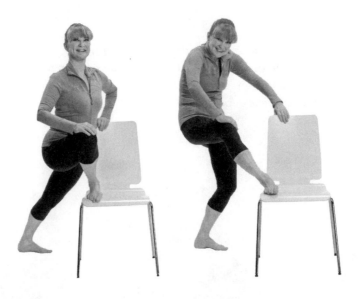

1. Face your chair and lift your knee straight to the ceiling.

2. Shift between rounding and straightening your back.

3. When you straighten your spine, shift the entire weight of your body forward toward the chair.

4. When you round your spine, shift your weight onto your back leg. As you shift from arch to straight, you will most likely find a tight spot. When you find a tight spot, slowly wiggle, trying to gently dislodge the blockage.

5. Repeat 4 times on both sides.

PSOAS AND QUADRICEPS CONNECTIVE TISSUE SEQUENCE

The psoas and quadriceps are called our hip flexors; they are essential for walking, sitting, and climbing stairs. When these muscles become unbalanced, the fascia of the psoas and quadriceps is impacted, blocking movement and causing injury and chronic pain. This two-phase exercise will stretch tight, unbalanced connective tissue in the psoas and quadriceps.

Phase One:

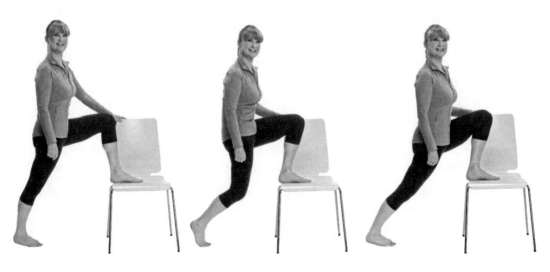

1. To begin the psoas stretch, hold the back of your chair and place one foot flat on the seat while you stand on your back leg (not too close to the chair).

2. Raise your back heel and bend your back knee, tucking under your lower spine.

3. Shift your weight forward toward the seat of the chair while keeping your body upright.

4. Try to straighten the back leg while pressing the back heel into the floor and maintaining the pelvic tuck. (To stretch the psoas muscles, it is necessary to keep your bum tucked under.)

5. Slowly repeat 3 times, then switch legs.

Phase Two:

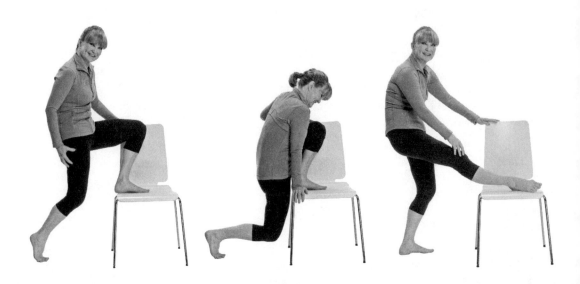

1. To begin the quadriceps stretch, stand at the side of your chair. Place one foot flat on the seat of the chair, while you stand on your back leg (not too close to the chair).

2. Holding the back of the chair for support, raise your back heel and bend your back knee, tucking under your lower spine.

3. Shift your weight forward toward the seat of the chair while keeping your body upright. Then relax your hips and try to touch the floor with your knee.

4. The moment you reach the depth of stretch you can comfortably support while remaining pain-free, straighten your back knee and come out of the stretch. Note: These movements are intended to be continuous and flowing; never hold a position longer than a few seconds.

5. Repeat this quadriceps stretch at least 3 times, then switch legs.

FULL-BODY CONNECTIVE TISSUE WINDMILL STRETCH

This sequence will stretch the fascia surrounding your hamstring muscles in addition to stretching your hips and spine. The large full-body movements in this sequence gently massage and loosen connective tissue in your legs and torso.

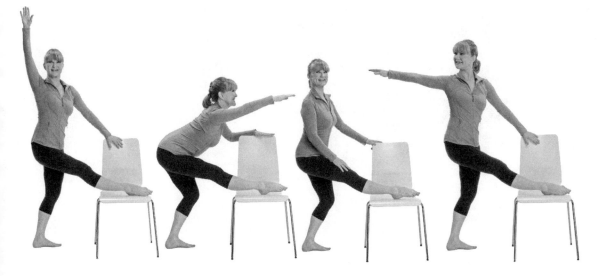

1. Stand beside your chair, holding the chair with one hand. Keep your standing knee slightly bent throughout the exercise. Place the leg farthest from the back of the chair on the seat of the chair and point your toe.

2. Lift that same arm above your head, and drop the hip down toward the ground. You will feel a stretch in your hamstrings and hips as you drop your hip.

3. Bend forward, keeping your spine straight while reaching over your leg; you will feel an immediate stretch in your hamstrings. (It is most important to keep your spine straight, so don't worry if you can barely bend forward—you will get more value out of the exercise if you keep your back straight in this section of the sequence.)

4. Gently sweep your arm toward the ground. Note: Your back will definitely round in this section, and you will feel a deeper stretch in your hamstrings.

5. Then sweep your arm behind you, rotating your spine toward the back of the room, turning as far as possible.

6. Finish the windmill by raising your arm above your head.

7. Repeat 3 to 4 arm windmills slowly on each leg.

Correct Modification for People with Tight Hamstrings

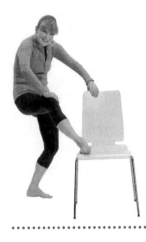

To keep the spine straight, bend both the standing leg and the leg on the chair.

Incorrect Modification for People with Tight Hamstrings

If your hamstrings are tight, do not round your back or tuck your tailbone under.

CHAPTER 12

The Immune System Workout

While still a teenager, Paula Hargraves got an up-close and personal look at lupus, a cruel, mysterious, and potentially fatal disease that affects about 1.5 million Americans, most of them women.

She and her future husband had just started dating when his stepmother was diagnosed with systemic lupus erythematosus (SLE). Paula witnessed the progression of the disease and saw the older woman beset by the side effects of medications along with heart, lung, and kidney disease. "I distinctly remember telling my husband that if I ever end up with an illness like that, I was not going to go the way she did," Paula said. "I wasn't going to just give up and be on the huge doses of prednisone and steroids and wait for the inevitable."

That memory served Paula well years later when she herself was diagnosed with SLE.

Lupus is an autoimmune disease—a function of the immune system attacking the body. Medical texts define SLE as a multisystemic disorder of connective tissue that proceeds through remissions and relapses. Lupus can be difficult to diagnose, especially if not caught early.

Lupus often hits people in the prime of their lives, and so it was with Paula. On a hiking trip with her husband in Nevada's Valley of Fire State Park to celebrate their tenth wedding anniversary, she found that her foot had become so swollen and painful that she could not walk, let alone hike the splendors of the park.

Over the course of close to a year, Paula was tested for everything from hairline bone fractures to sexually transmitted diseases to heart problems. "It was horrible and it just kept getting worse and worse and worse," she said. She had flulike symptoms, digestive problems, and chronic urinary tract infections. The pain was spreading into her joints, and she lost her flexibility.

At the time, Paula had a corporate job in downtown San Francisco, and she needed to be at work at eight every morning. She lived across the Bay in Oakland and commuted by the regional rail service. Without a diagnosis, she was relying on over-the-counter ibuprofen for pain relief and, she added, lots of caffeine to get through the day. During this time she became beset by fainting spells.

It was difficult at work for Paula but hellish commuting. To ensure she got a seat on the train in case she felt faint, she rose extra early to catch the train going up the line, away from San Francisco. Climbing stairs or taking escalators was slow and painful. Once when she fell on an escalator, no one came to her aid.

Finally, Paula was diagnosed with hypothyroidism—a condition in which an underactive thyroid gland doesn't produce enough of certain important hormones—as well as SLE. Paula was thirty-six years old and devastated to learn she had the disease that had consumed her husband's stepmother. She had also been diagnosed with Sjögren's syndrome (a little-known autoimmune disorder that can accompany lupus and whose symptoms include joint pain and a general feeling of body fatigue); Raynaud's phenomenon (a condition which causes body areas such as fingers and toes to feel numb and cold); and fibromyalgia (a pain-amplification syndrome that afflicts six million Americans and is characterized by chronic neuromuscular pain, widespread stiffness, and aching). In less than six years, Paula's life had become a hardscrabble existence dominated by illness and pain.

"I had been a field biologist at one point—I was used to hiking up sides of mountains, birding, walking, doing dance and yoga," she recalled. "I went from being very active, very outdoors-oriented . . . to barely being able to walk across a parking lot."

The first rheumatologist who treated her was remarkably unsympathetic and barely acknowledged her pain. Paula recalled, "I would tell him, I have such terrible pain, I'm barely functioning. He said, 'Well, you should see some of my patients. They are almost dying. You can't complain.'"

As it is, Paula says she is the only person still alive among the lupus sufferers she knew when she was diagnosed with the disease. "One poor girl was only sixteen or seventeen years old. Another was a woman in her early thirties who had two young children, a terrible tragedy," Paula said. "I was lucky that when I was first diagnosed, I had no organ involvement."

Once diagnosed, Paula decided that she was going to do everything she could to regain her health. Reflecting on the experience of her husband's stepmother, she decided to fight hard. "You really have to harness your own inner strength and sense of survival," she said, "and the idea that you want to be better in order to move yourself forward, to be better."

Paula found a few allies among health-care providers, notably her personal physician and a second—more helpful—rheumatologist. But in the wider world, she felt isolated by her illness and the pain that would flare from manageable to horrendous without warning. She couldn't do ordinary things like go out to dinner with friends because she never knew how she'd feel or whether the pain would kick up to the sobbing-on-the-floor level. Friends slowly drifted away.

"My acupuncturist, who is also my physician, always called these autoimmune illnesses the hidden illnesses because people look at you and think you are fine because you don't look like you are on death's door. In movies, they make people look really, really sick when they are 'ill' so that they appear 'ill' on camera . . . but many people who are really ill don't appear outwardly ill until they are very far down the path of their illness," she said.

Paula says she learned to mask her illness and say she was feeling fine when asked about her health even though the pain levels were what she called excruciatingly high. In the privacy of her home, she'd joke to her husband that the only thing that didn't hurt was the tip of her nose. In public, though, things were not always funny. When she would say she had lupus, most people had no idea what that was. "Once," she recalled, "someone at work asked me how I was doing and I said, 'Well, I'm managing but there is a lot of pain; there is never any time that I don't hurt.' And that person said to me, 'Oh well, just be glad you don't have cancer.' I thought that that was not only such a noncompassionate thing to say, but also it really showed that people don't understand what it is like to have an auto-immune illness."

Some things got gradually better for Paula. She took a short-term disability leave from work, which helped her come to terms with her illness while building up the fortitude to return to the job part-time.

She and her husband strategically moved to a warmer, drier region in the Bay Area, where there were fewer storms. The better climate lessened the bouts of "horrendous" pain related to shifts in barometric pressure. Her new rheumatologist was open to alternative treatments and complementary medicine such as Chinese herbs, the practice of qigong, and treatments from a chiropractor.

Paula says her biggest leap in the right direction occurred in 2007 when she happened on *Classical Stretch* and the Essentrics exercise program. "It was one of those days when I was really, really sick and couldn't make it to work and was too ill to eat," she recalled. "I was channel-surfing on PBS and happened, just by chance, to come across your program." By the time Paula could rouse herself from the couch where she had been lying, the episode was nearing its end.

"I did the rest of the program as best I could. I was terribly, terribly stiff at the time, in pain and ill that day. But at the end, I felt better and thought, 'This is great!'" Paula decided to record the episodes to do them on the weekend. "Then I realized it would help me get through the day better," she said, "so I made the commitment to get up a half hour earlier to exercise before I went to work. Initially, it was hard . . . but when I started doing the program regularly, I found that I was sleeping better."

Stubbornness and persistence helped offset the daily frustration of not being able to do the exercises as well as she wanted. Paula recalled, "I just kept with it. I wasn't able to do it normally. I couldn't keep up. I had to move very slowly. I didn't have the strength to do many arm exercises. I couldn't do leg lifts for a long time. The pliés were very difficult. Any strengthening of the back was very difficult. I would just have to go slow, sometimes skip parts. I just did it in a very relaxed state and to the best of my ability every time."

Paula says that within about six months, she was able to do the complete program. At that point, she was doing Essentrics every day unless something extraordinary like a trip out of town prevented it.

Paula decided to leave her high-pressure job, which created too much stress for her compromised system to handle. She has focused on nutrition, switching to a vegan diet, which she says helps her manage her pain levels. While she still suffers from the occasional flare-ups, she's doing better than ever.

"I can absolutely say that this exercise program has cured me of the fibromyalgia," says Paula. "I've never had that kind of pain again."

In our muscles, mechanoreceptors—sense organs that respond to mechanical stimuli such as pressure or sound—both gather information about the full body's health and send that information to the brain through muscle movement. This information is used to feed the immune system with information, thereby stimulating and strengthening it. I believe this is why correct alignment and full-body movement played a major role in strengthening and regulating Paula's immune system. Good alignment helps recruit all muscles, allowing them to gather massive amounts of information that the brain feeds back to the immune system. The more we use our muscles, the stronger the organs become. In Paula's case, good alignment and full-body movements might be partly why she is winning the battle with her immune system as she faithfully exercises on a daily basis. We should never underestimate our own body's ability to self-heal given the correct environment.

Muscles are made of trillions of protein fibers that slide in and out of spaghetti-shaped cells. When the sliding action is prevented from happening, the result is pain from a scale of mild to excruciating to unbearable. A neurological disorder like fibromyalgia damages the essential sliding action of our muscle fibers, leading to a cascade of chronic pain-related conditions, including neurological conditions like back spasms, charley horses, fibromyalgia, and lupus. Pain will strike if the muscle fibers are locked in spasm because the message to release the contraction is not reaching the fibers. Spasm is a hallmark symptom of fibromyalgia, and it endangers muscle health, leading to muscle fiber damage. In healthy, pain-free muscles, there is a constant automatic interplay between contraction and relaxation of the muscle fibers. But with spasm, the automatic message is interrupted and the muscle is incapable of relaxing on its own. At that point, we have to physically pull out the contraction with exercise. Eccentric stretching pulls on the contracted muscle cells, releasing the spasm, relieving the danger of cell damage, and—best of all—ending the pain.

To address the pain of spasm from fibromyalgia and strengthen an immune system weakened by lupus, we need a vibrant muscular skeletal system. Every muscular skeletal system requires regular full-body rebalancing, aligning, stretching, and strengthening exercises to become and remain healthy and pain-free. Essentrics and tai chi are fitness programs that stretch, strengthen, realign, and rebalance the entire skeletal musculature, achieving the goals of spasm release and full-body rebalancing.

SIDE-TO-SIDE WINDOW WASHES FOR IMMUNITY

The spine is designed to bend in many directions. This exercise will increase the flexibility and strength of the obliques (the side muscles of the abdomen) and the rib muscles that support your spine, helping to make everyday movements, such as dressing, brushing hair, or cooking, easy and pain-free. The side-to-side bends rebalance the spinal musculature and relieve pain.

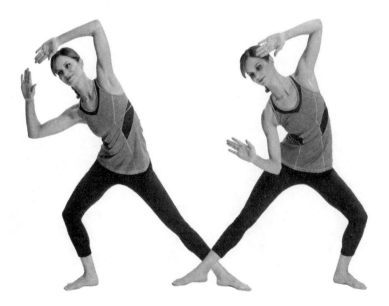

1. Start in a side lunge, bending sideways with your arms framing your head and your elbows bent.

2. Imagine you are standing very close to a window while you are washing it. Open your fingers as wide as possible throughout the exercise.

3. Keep your elbows bent and your forearms beside your ears as you wash the window, sweeping across your body.

4. Shift your ribs, feeling a stretch in them as you bend your torso while lunging side to side.

5. Throughout this sequence, imagine that you are pressed between two plates of glass, one in front of you and one behind; this image will help you keep your back straight and upright. Imagine that you have a wide rag in your hands; that will help you keep your hands flat on the imaginary window as you drag them across.

6. When you have bent as far as you can, change sides; let your torso sway sideways as you change sides.

7. Alternate sides with each wash at least 8 times, and don't stop between each side—keep flowing from one side to the next.

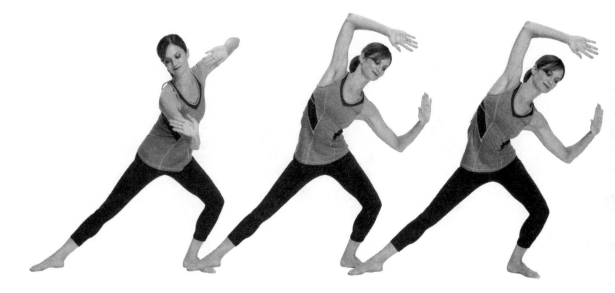

> **Modification Note:**
>
> To make the exercise more strengthening: Imagine that you are washing a sticky substance off a window. This will make your muscles contract as you move.
>
> To make the exercise easier: Imagine you are wiping the window with a silk cloth. This will keep your muscles relaxed.

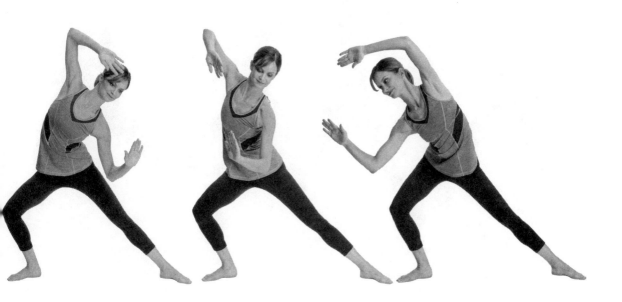

FULL-BODY STRAIGHT-ARM FIGURE 8 SEQUENCE

Many of the shoulder muscles can be engaged, stretched, and strengthened only when using a straight arm. This figure 8 sequence works every muscle, from the fingertips, through the entire spine, down the legs, and into the feet. It pulls apart tight locked muscles and joints, giving rapid relief to areas where the muscles have been blocked from moving.

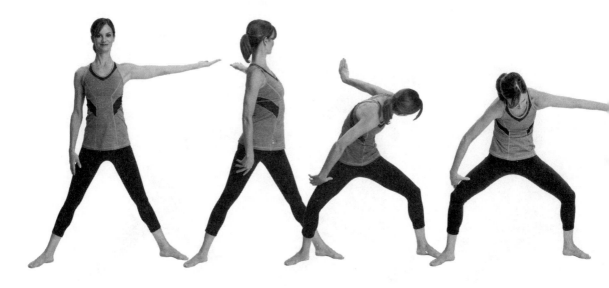

1. Stand with your feet comfortably wide apart; extend one arm to shoulder height, keeping the other relaxed by your side.

2. Rotate your spine, twisting your extended arm behind you, and look behind you.

3. Bend slightly forward as you bend your knees, tuck your pelvis under, and gently rotate your twisted arm within your shoulder socket.

4. Continue looking behind you while turning slightly to the back.

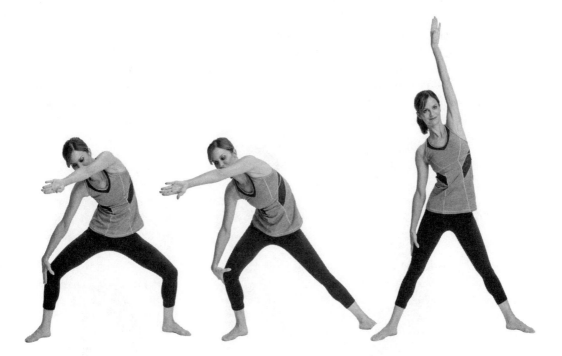

5. Return your torso to face the front and slowly sweep your rotated arm across your body—keep it rotated in your shoulder socket the entire time. This will pull through the entire musculature of your shoulder girdle and into your back muscles.

6. Shift your weight into a deep side lunge while sweeping the arm across your body.

7. Then raise your arm above your head and straighten your legs.

8. Repeat the entire sequence 3 to 4 times before alternating sides.

REBALANCING SPINE SEQUENCE

This exercise is an amazing sequence for rebalancing the entire torso: spine, abdominal, and gluteus muscles. Back pain is often caused when the torso's muscles become un-balanced: too weak, too strong, or too tight. This sequence will unlock the muscles of your spine, ribs, and hips, liberating compressed, damaged joints. While following these exercises, focus on the full spine: the front and back. Imagine as you are doing the exercise that you are using every one of your thirty-three vertebrae separately.

If some parts of your spine are blocked and won't budge, which is common, don't give up. Keep trying. Don't focus on being perfect but instead, focus on feeling any movement at all along your spine. Even the tiniest movement means that you are slowly unlocking your joints and muscles. Over time, they will loosen up.

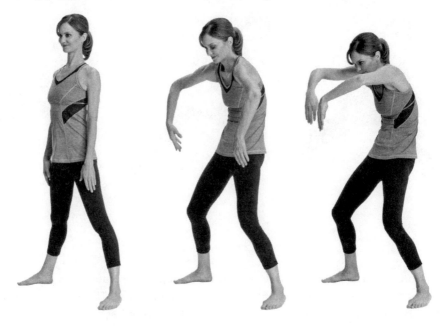

1. Stand straight with your feet apart and arms at your sides.

2. Bend your knees, tuck your tailbone under, round your back, and raise your shoulders.

3. Lift your arms in front to shoulder height, keeping them relaxed.

4. Lift your shoulders as high as possible.

5. Reverse the position by standing straight and lifting your arms over your head as you open your chest.

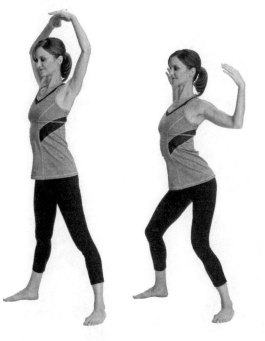

6. Pull your arms behind you, keeping your elbows bent and lowering your shoulders. Imagine that you are slipping your shoulder blades into your back pockets.

7. At the same time, bend your knees and arch your back by sticking out your bum.

8. Return to starting position.

9. Repeat this sequence slowly at least 8 times in a row.

• •

Incorrect Spine Position in Rebalancing Sequence

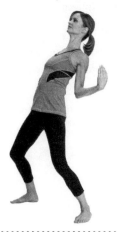

Do not lean backward in this sequence. Dropping backward will push your body weight forward, stressing your knees and compressing your lower vertebrae.

• •

THIGHS, KNEES, AND FINGERS

This sequence will relieve compression while also strengthening and stretching wrists and fingers. Pain in the quadriceps, hips, and fingers is common among fibromyalgia sufferers.

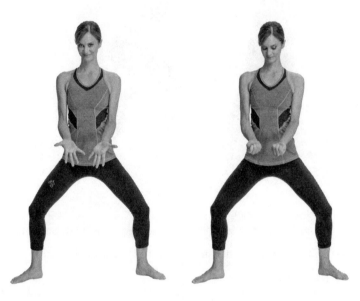

1. Stand in a wide tai chi stance, with your feet much wider than your hips. Line up the thighbone with your feet to ensure clean alignment and no torsion on the ankles.

2. Keep your back straight during the entire exercise.

3. Count to 5 as you bend your knees into the plié. Remain in the bent-knee plié position as long as you can, strengthening the gluteus muscles and quadriceps, while doing the hand and finger part of this exercise.

4. Open and close your hands, stretching and extending the fingers as much as possible.

5. Repeat opening and closing the hands 4 times before straightening your legs. (Repeat no more than 4 times.)

HIP CLEANERS FOR IMMUNITY

The purpose of hip cleaners is to remove dead or congealed tissue that leads to stiffness and poor hip mobility. The rotational movement of the thighbone in the hip socket performs a sloughing action within the socket. Often what we think are stiff muscles are really joints that are gummed up. These hip cleaners will give you a whole sense of new energy and mobility.

While doing this exercise, try not to move your hips—focus on rotating your leg within the hip socket. During the exercise, try to relax your hips and knees. Never stop to hold a position; keep moving in a smooth, fluid motion.

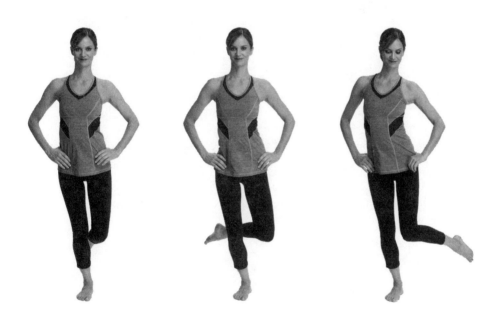

1. Begin by lifting one leg with the knee bent behind you.

2. Swing the bent leg slightly behind your other leg.

3. Lift your bent leg higher and rotate the thigh internally in the hip socket. (You will notice that the foot will automatically swing to the outside.)

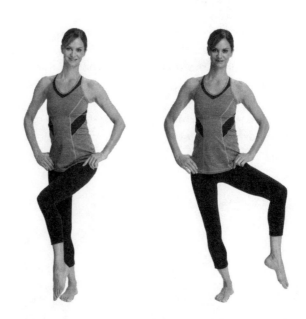

4. Draw the knee diagonally in front of your body; you will feel a stretch in your bum. Note: While doing this exercise, hold the hips still as you rotate the leg within the hip-socket.

5. Lift the bent leg higher and, drawing it across the front of the body, open the leg as wide as possible to the side.

6. Return to the starting position

7. Repeat 4 to 8 times per leg.

NEUROLOGICAL HIP STRETCH

The hip-blast sequence employs the neurological technique called proprioceptive neuromuscular facilitation (PNF), which involves muscle contraction, release, and stretch. (See the box on page 135.) The PNF will give you an amazing feeling of freedom in your hips.

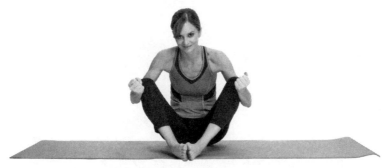

1. Sit on the ground with your knees bent and the soles of your feet touching comfortably in front of you.

2. Lift your knees and hold them tightly with your arms, and then try to force your knees toward the floor. The trick here is to block your knees from lowering. This will create a buildup of tension in the groin (or hip region, depending on the person).

3. Let go of your knees and try to relax your hips and groin for 2 or 3 seconds

4. Hold your shins just above your ankles and bend forward, placing your elbows on your knees.

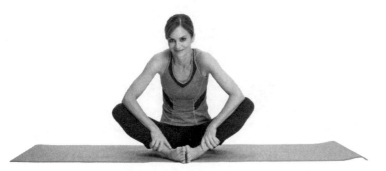

5. Bend forward, using your elbows to push down on your knees; you will feel a strong stretch in your groin or hips.

6. Repeat the sequence 3 or 4 times slowly.

REBALANCING HIP AND GROIN SEQUENCE

This old-school gym favorite, done the Essentrics way, is great for targeting and lengthening shortened groin muscles. Doing these every day will also further help open and relieve pressure on the hip joints.

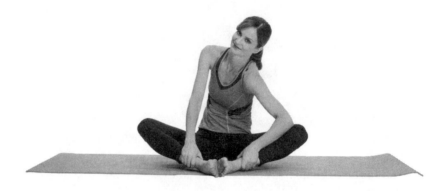

1. Sit comfortably (your back can be rounded), holding your shins just above your ankles.

2. Place one elbow on one knee and gently press down on the knee; you will feel a stretch in one groin muscle.

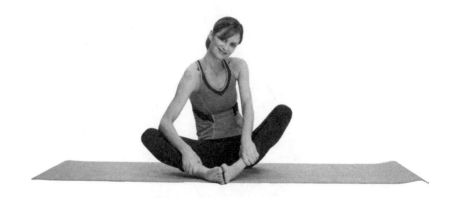

3. Hold for about 6 seconds, then change to the other knee and stretch the other groin muscle.

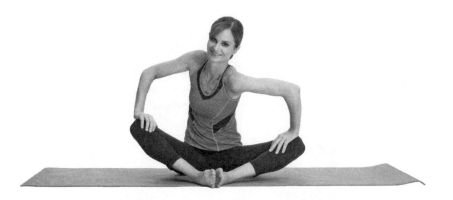

4. Repeat 4 times, alternating sides each time.

5. Add on a deeper stretch by placing your hands on either knee and gently pressing down on your knee. Hold this deep stretch for 6 seconds, then release the pressure.

6. Repeat 4 times, alternating sides each time.

SIDE LEG LIFTS

Side leg lifts strengthen the short inner muscles of the hips. I have heard from many people suffering from fibromyalgia that these exercises help relieve spasm by stretching and strengthening the hips. Even though they primarily target the hips, they strengthen the entire leg as well as the obliques and the spinal muscles.

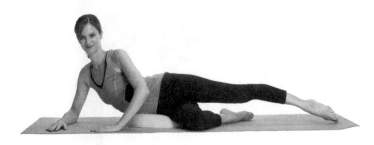

1. Start by placing a hemorrhoid cushion on your mat, and lie on your side with your hip in the hole of the cushion.

2. Bend your lower leg and keep your upper leg straight.

3. Keep your weight tilted slightly forward—don't allow your body to rock or fall backward.

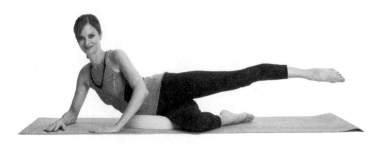

4. Slowly lift and then lower your leg while imagining that you are pulling your leg out of your hip socket (and reach toward the wall).

5. Keep your movements slow and controlled; lifting quickly uses momentum and will not strengthen or stretch your muscle. (If you are properly pulling your leg out of your

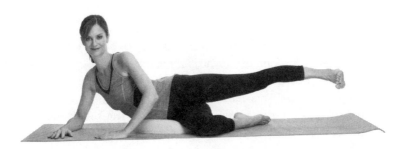

hip socket, you should not be able to lift it any higher than Sahra does in the photo above.)

6. Repeat 8 to 16 times with a pointed foot and then 8 to 16 times with a flexed foot.

7. Switch sides and repeat the same sequence with the opposite leg.

REBALANCING HAMSTRING STRETCH

The hamstring muscles cross two joints; they start on our hipbone and finish by attaching to our shinbone. Located on the back side of our leg, opposite from our quadriceps, the hamstrings are one of the largest muscle groups in our body. When they are tight and stiff, they pull the hipbone close to the thighbone, squeezing the joint and causing joint compression. This causes us to lose our range of motion when walking and running, and even making sitting painful and difficult. This rebalancing hamstring stretch will loosen the tension, therefore decompressing the joint and relieving hip pain.

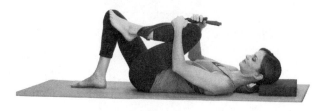

1. Lie flat on your back, with your spine and hips flat on the ground.
2. Bend one leg, keeping the foot flat on the ground.

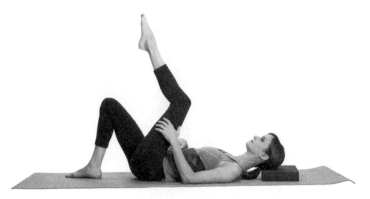

3. Raise the other leg, bending the knee of that leg. Hold the knee with both hands and pull it toward your chest.
4. While doing this, relax your bum and wiggle it under you. (The wiggling of the bum will force the hip muscle to relax, making the next movement easier to do.)
5. Release your hold on the knee, raise your leg higher, and try to straighten the knee. Note: If your hamstrings are tight, you may not be able to straighten your knee completely; in that case, leave it slightly bent.

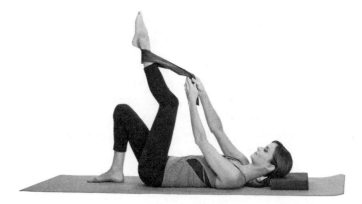

6. Wrap a stretch band comfortably around your lower leg, near your ankle. Use the band to pull your leg toward your chest while keeping your head flat on the floor.

7. Using the PNF techniques, resist with a push, release, relax more with the wiggle, and then pull again.

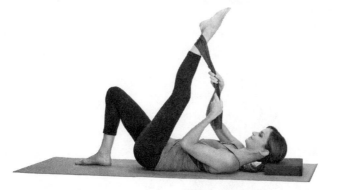

8. Push against the band, trying to lower your leg toward the floor. (The band will stop you from being able to lower your leg too far.) Push for 3 to 6 seconds.

9. Stop pushing against the band and relax your hips for 3 seconds.

10. Wiggle your bum for 3 seconds.

11. Using the band, pull the leg toward your chest again. (The band will help you deepen the stretch.) Hold for about 6 seconds.

12. Relax 6 seconds before starting again.

13. Repeat 3 times before changing legs.

QUADRICEPS SEQUENCE

This quadriceps stretch is popular with people who are suffering from fibromyalgia. It stretches unseen muscle chains that run through the entire body. Some people find the seated position in this exercise, awkward. If you are not comfortable doing this exercise, it's perfectly fine to skip it—you decide. The Thighs, Knees, and Fingers exercises in this chapter (see page 216) also stretch and strengthen the quadriceps.

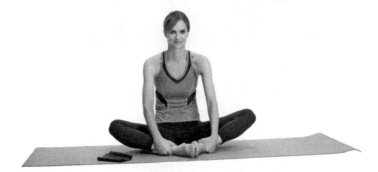

1. Sit on the ground with your knees bent and the soles of your feet together.

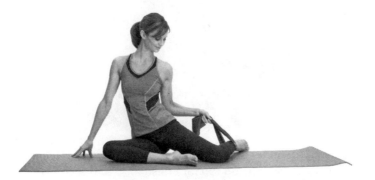

2. Gently rotate one leg behind you. Wrap a stretch band around your back ankle. Make sure your thigh muscles are higher than your knee and that your knee joint is not touching the ground. Note: Never put the weight of your body directly on the knee joint. This could easily damage the patella—that is, your kneecap—and the cartilage of the joint.

3. Pull the band toward your bum, which will gently pull your ankle toward you. (You should feel a stretch in your quadriceps.)

4. Hold the stretch for 6 seconds.

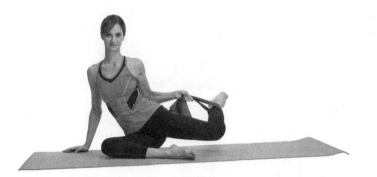

5. Stop pulling toward you with band and, instead, *push* your leg against the band. (You should feel a contraction in your quadriceps.)

6. Hold the contraction for 6 seconds.

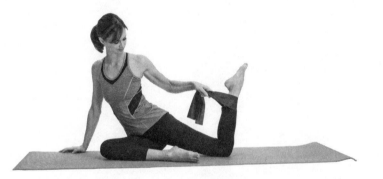

7. Start again by pulling the ankle toward your bum with the stretch band.

8. Repeat the entire sequence 3 times on each leg.

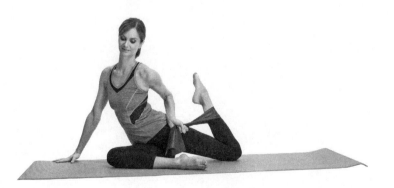

CHAPTER 13

The Arthritis Workout

Annick Daigle was ten weeks shy of her thirty-fourth birthday when her doctor gave her the grim news: she had rheumatoid arthritis. "The doctor told me, 'Pain is going to be part of your life from now on. You'd better learn how to cope with that,'" she said. It was a chilling message for an active and ambitious young woman just starting to hit her stride in the physically demanding and male-dominated railroad industry. "Pain becomes a partner in your life whether you want it or not," the now fifty-one-year-old Annick recalled.

She experienced her first taste of arthritic pain in college, when her fingers would throb every time she wrote out lengthy responses to exam questions. But in the two years prior to her diagnosis, the pain had escalated. She often couldn't get out of bed without feeling what she called awful pain. The only way she could manage was to roll out and land on her hands and knees before slowly standing up, one vertebra at a time.

When Annick discusses her disease, she talks about how lucky she has been compared with others with arthritis. A prime example of her good fortune, she says, was finding a skilled rheumatologist who gave her—along with the proper medications—wise counsel about the need to prepare for the challenge of chronic pain and the need to exercise. She was also diagnosed at an early stage. The medication prescribed to her was effective enough to essentially put the disease on hold for about eight years. Annick considers that plateau in the illness, a period that was essentially pain-free, a most wonderful gift.

And then one day the medication suddenly stopped working; Annick's condition worsened and pain started to roam her body, moving from joint to joint. It woke her up at night, made her cranky and short-tempered and, most problematic, limited how she lived, worked, and played. Annick had officially joined millions of people worldwide who suffer daily from the enduring stiffness, swelling, and pain of rheumatoid arthritis.

Arthritis, a condition that causes severe joint damage and pain, can strike suddenly without warning or sneak up slowly. It is one of the most common health conditions in the world, and it is currently the number one cause of disability in the United States: more than 50 million adults and 300,000 children have some type of arthritis, according to the Arthritis Foundation. There are more than one hundred different types. The most common form is osteoarthritis, a degenerative joint disease. A less common form is rheumatoid arthritis, an autoimmune disease in which the body's immune system mistakenly attacks the joints.

For the eight years between Annick's diagnosis of arthritis and the onset of her chronic pain, she felt good. During that period, Annick worked for one of North America's leading railroad companies. When the company announced it was looking for new trainmasters, Annick applied and got the position.

The job was—and still is—physically demanding. The position of trainmaster is a critical frontline supervisory position best suited for those who thrive under pressure. Annick rose to the challenge. In her junior years as a trainmaster, she was put in charge of the fourteen-hour night shifts. It was under those conditions that her initial arthritis medication stopped being effective.

She and her doctor settled on other effective medication, but the disease escalated again. She was now living with chronic pain. Her doctor suggested that Annick use over-the-counter pain medication, up to the maximum daily dosage. She became proactive about pain control, taking Tylenol if she knew she would be doing a lot of physical work or if weather conditions and humidity levels were such that she knew pain was in her forecast. However, she wasn't as proactive with her nutrition.

"Diet-wise, as a trainmaster, I ate the worst of my life," Annick recalled. The many years of poor nutrition did nothing to strengthen her already embattled immune system. Annick realizes now how important a healthy diet is to her immune system, but at the time it was not something her doctor talked about. "I was young and loving my job," she said. "I sacrificed a balanced diet, not thinking of possible health consequences down the road."

As the pain got worse, Annick developed various ways of coping with it. "When I have a severe arthritis attack my hands can't move, my elbows can't bend, all my joints can't move," she explained. "I can't even take big breaths, just shallow breaths. I have trouble breathing because the rib cage is attached to the spine, and when you breathe, the ribs move with the breath whether you want them to or not. When you expand the rib cage to breathe in, all those little vertebrae hurt like crazy. Sometimes the pain is a twelve on the scale of one to ten," she says. Those occasions are relatively rare now—but Annick knows that her disease will progress. She takes full advantage of the latest technology available to help arthritis sufferers. One device she finds particularly helpful is a transcutaneous electrical nerve stimulation (TENS) unit, which generates painless, low-level electric impulses that stimulate certain nerves. It is thought that TENS may trigger the release of endorphins and may also block nerve pathways that carry pain messages. Annick also started a daily practice of meditation accompanied by regularly practicing qigong, a form of meditation and exercise. Both helped her develop the resilience she needed to accept pain as a constant in her life. "When you can't control pain, it controls you. That was something that was difficult for me to accept because I'm a bit of a control freak," she said. "Meditation helped me be more zen about life, about not being disturbed by something I can't control."

A couple of years ago, over her Christmas break, Annick happened to watch the *Aging Backwards* documentary on her local PBS station. "It struck a chord," she said. When she sought out more information, Annick was amazed to learn that there was an Essentrics studio within walking distance of her office.

That's when her life changed. After six months of regular Essentrics workouts, her pain began to subside. "After the first class, I said, 'This is it. I've finally found it,'" Annick recalled. The stretching and strengthening aspect of that first class opened up her body in unexpected ways, relieving her of pain immediately. She told a friend, "It feels like I have more space inside of me. I feel like my organs have been moved around and I have more breathing space. I don't know exactly what, but something has happened."

Annick is convinced that Essentrics has helped reduce her chronic pain. "My posture is better, the way I walk is better, it probably helps the joint pain because I'm better aligned," she explained. "It might be all just psychological. I don't really care why, but yes, I can tell you, it has helped me reduce pain tremendously. Even my mood is better. I feel like the energy we all have inside of us is flowing again."

Essentrics helped Annick with her chronic pain for many reasons. Pulling the joints "open" offered immediate relief from the constant compression of inflamed joints rubbing together. The pulling apart of joints is the definition of what an eccentric movement is; Essentrics simultaneously strengthens and stretches the muscles. This technique also lubricates congealed joints in the same way that moving a door joint while oiling the hinge distributes the lubrication through the hinge more effectively, helping the door swing more smoothly.

Essentrics also stimulates the release of endorphins, our natural endogenous opioids, which have many beneficial qualities, including improvement of mood, relief of pain, and increase in energy. Annick commented on an improvement in these three symptoms.

Because Essentrics is a relatively slow-moving workout, it allows you to go to your personal limit and stop when movements become painful or uncomfortable. The slow pace has two advantages: it removes the fear of hurting yourself while exercising, and it prevents injuries. These two qualities are essential in gaining strength and flexibility. Gaining additional strength is a major side benefit of moving slowly versus using momentum. The slower you go, the more your muscles are required to accomplish the movement, which naturally increases your strength. When you move rapidly, you use momentum; not only does it not require strength, it damages your joints and can inflame or increase the chances of tearing sensitive tissues.

By using movements that flow through all the muscle and connective-tissue chains of the body, Essentrics stimulates a powerful flood of messages from all the major muscle, neurological, and connective tissue chains to the brain and into the immune system. The combination of correct full-body exercises, muscle strengthening, and bone alignment together are the most powerful trio to stimulate and feed the immune system. All autoimmune conditions, such as rheumatoid arthritis, can benefit from this improved communication between the major systems of our body.

———

This workout is for all arthritis sufferers. Osteoarthritis, the most common type of arthritis, is identified by joint degeneration; it is caused by muscle imbalance and regular impact on the joint. As you do this workout, try to keep your body in a constant state of motion. Don't hold any of the movements in positions or poses—keep moving through the sequences. The constant motion will help lubricate your joints. Moving slowly and easily should leave you feeling relaxed and pain-free when the sequence is finished. Make sure to have a chair nearby for support.

The initial pain of osteoarthritis indicates that degeneration is starting, but stretching and strengthening the joint can help stop the damage and relieve the pain. However, if the degeneration has gone unchecked for a long time, the joint may be too severely degenerated to be healed through exercise alone. Even if the pain is relieved through exercise, it doesn't mean the arthritis has been reversed.

Essentrics helps relieve the pain of arthritis because it strengthens the muscles in a lengthened position, literally pulling the joints apart. In separating the joints, the intense grinding of bone on bone is stopped, and the pain disappears. No actual healing has taken place, only the relief of pain. The squeezing and compressing of the joints is what causes the grinding damage of arthritis. When the compressing and squeezing stop, so does the pain.

CEILING REACHES FOR ARTHRITIS

This simple exercise will rebalance your muscles, realign your spine, and decompress your vertebrae by stretching and strengthening your back muscles. When we stretch and strengthen the joints of the spine, we relieve arthritic pain.

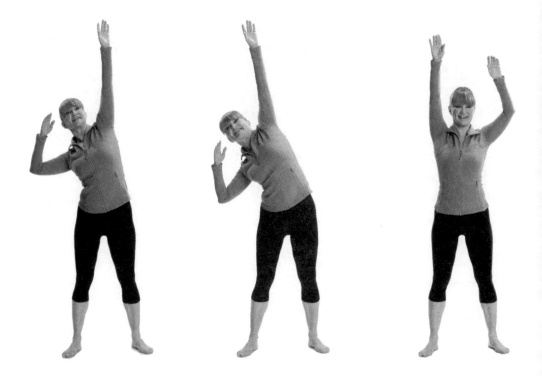

1. Start in an open stance with your feet apart.

2. Raise one arm to the ceiling, and count to 3 while trying to pull it higher.

3. Contract the shoulder muscles and count to 3, holding the contraction as tightly as you can.

4. Completely relax the shoulder muscles; take a few seconds to feel the muscles letting go of the contraction.

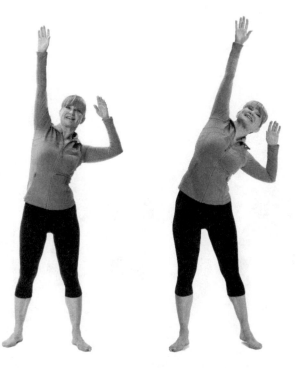

5. When your shoulder muscles are fully relaxed, again count to 3 while reaching higher toward the ceiling; feel the shoulder joint open up as it relaxes.

6. Keep your arm above your head and repeat the whole contract-relax-reach sequence 3 times.

7. Change arms and repeat the entire series on the other side. Note: You can repeat these ceiling reaches as many times as you like and as often during the day as you choose. They are safe to do as often as you want.

FULL-BODY WAIST ROTATIONS

To liberate your joints, you need to strengthen the muscles while they are in a lengthened position. In the full-body waist rotations, the thirty-three vertebrae of the spine are both stretched and strengthened. These continuous rotations force the blood to circulate throughout the spine, hips, and legs, nourishing the bones by delivering calcium, oxygen, and other essential nutrients. These rotations engage virtually every muscle in the body from fingers to toes.

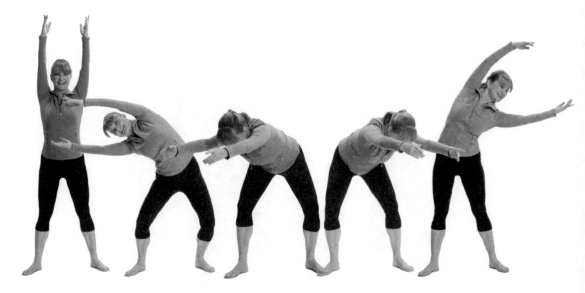

1. Stand with your feet apart in a position that is comfortably wider than your hips.

2. Lift your arms above your head. Throughout the exercise, try to keep your arms as close to each other as possible, with your elbows straight (if you can) and your arms next to your ears (again if you can). Note: Very tight triceps and pectoral muscles can make this difficult. If you find it impossible to keep your elbows straight, bend them. If you find it impossible to keep them in line with your ears, lower them. Work on straightening your elbows and raising your arms to the correct height each time you exercise.

3. Bend your knees and slowly bend your entire body sideways, extending your spine into as long a length as possible while moving.

4. Tuck your tailbone under, round your spine, and rotate your torso toward the floor while keeping your arms beside your ears. Do these rotations as slowly as possible throughout the exercise. Note: Whenever you bend forward, always be sure to tuck your tailbone under. This will protect your spine from becoming overloaded and stressed.

5. Remain in motion as you slowly sweep your body to the other side.

6. Rotate your torso to face the front, while bending sideways and straightening your knees.

7. Finish in the same upright position in which you started.

8. Reverse direction and repeat 2 to 4 rotations, alternating direction each time.

Incorrect Spine in Waist Rotations

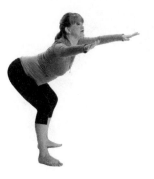

Don't stick out your bum or maintain a straight spine when bending forward—always tuck your tailbone under. Keeping the bum out in this spine rotation will put stress on your lower spine, overloading your muscles and compressing your vertebrae.

SIDE-TO-SIDE LUNGES

This sequence will stretch and strengthen the muscles of your spine, liberating rigid locked vertebrae. It will prevent damage to the vertebrae and relieve present joint pain.

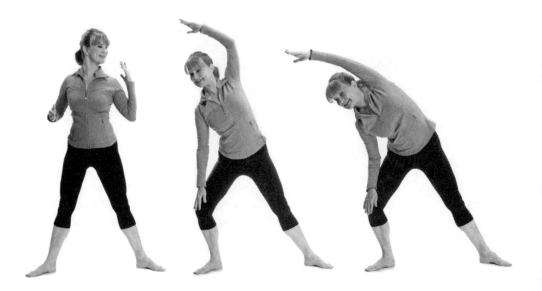

1. Stand in a wide stance with one arm bent and your hand almost touching your shoulder.

2. Extend that arm over your head while you lunge to the opposite side.

3. Progressively deepen the side bend as you reach the extended arm toward the wall.

4. Shift your weight to your other leg as you prepare to repeat the lunge on the other side.

5. As you shift your weight from one leg to the other, keep your knees in line with your feet and be careful not to let your knees drop forward. (When your knees drop forward, the joint twists, leading to damage and pain.)

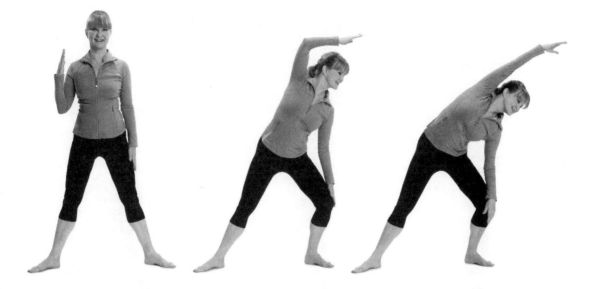

6. As you raise one arm, let the other arm relax by your side. Follow the side of your body with your arm, bending the elbow and straightening it as you do the deep side stretch.

7. With every side-to-side lunge, bend sideways as far as you can before changing sides.

8. Repeat the side-to-side lunges 16 times, slowly alternating sides.

···

Incorrect Posture for a Side Bend

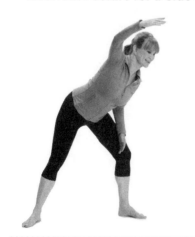

Do not lift your hips as you bend your torso sideways. If you lift your hips, the muscles will not be stretched, and stretching is what liberates the vertebrae and relieves spinal pain.

···

DIAGONAL LUNGES

These diagonal lunges rebalance the full skeleton, liberating all the joints in the body.

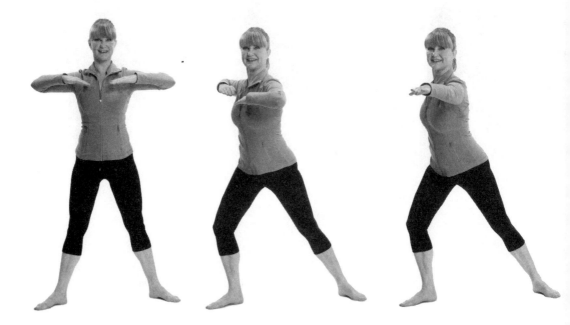

1. Stand in a wide stance, elbows bent and arms at shoulder height.

2. Without changing the position of your feet, turn your hips slightly toward one side and bend the knee on that side, shifting into a front lunge.

3. Rotate the torso and extend your arm diagonally in front of your body.

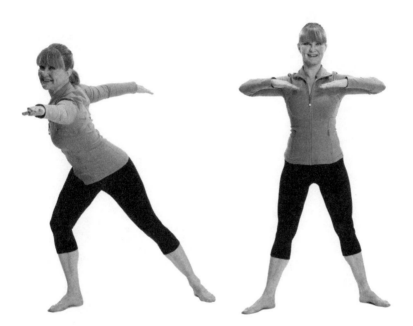

4. As you lunge deeper, rotate your torso as much as possible while reaching forward with your front arm and backward with the other.

5. Keep your spine straight while bending over your front leg.

6. Return to your starting position.

7. Repeat, alternating sides, 8 to 16 times.

HANDS, FINGERS, AND WRISTS

The most common locations of pain for arthritis suffers are fingers/hands/wrists and ankles/toes/feet. You can do these hand exercises as often as you'd like during the day; they are safe and will bring immediate relief. The more often you do them and the harder you work at opening and closing your hands, working individual fingers, and rotating your wrists, the faster you will feel results. You will see a significant reduction in arthritic pain if you do these exercises on a regular basis.

Phase One:

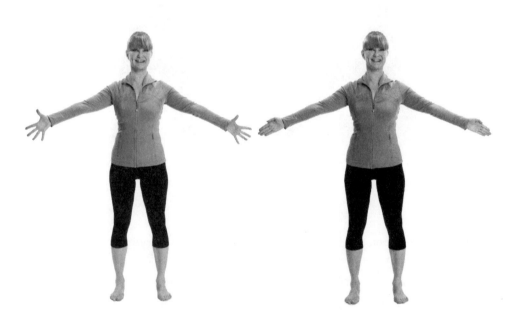

1. Stand with your feet apart and your arms reaching out to either side with your hands open.

2. Spread your fingers as wide as possible.

3. When you have spread them to your maximum, try spreading them more!

4. Close your fingers tightly together.

5. Repeat 16 times slowly and 16 times rapidly.

Phase Two:

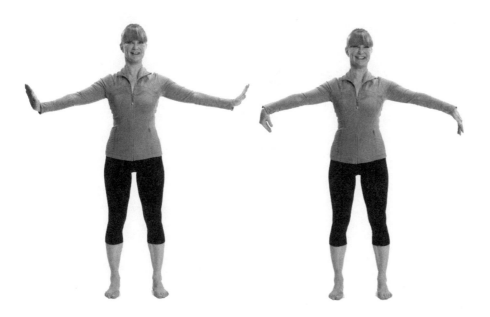

1. With flat palms, extend your hands and rotate them within your wrists, drawing a circle.

2. Repeat slowly.

3. Draw 4 circles in each direction.

Phase Three:

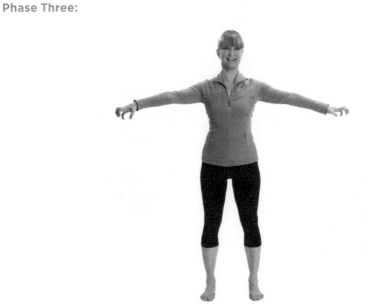

1. With your arms outstretched, imagine that you are playing the piano with bent fingers.

2. Keep your arms straight while you move your fingers as rapidly as possible over the imaginary piano keys for about 1 minute. (Play some piano music while doing this finger exercise to inspire you.)

3. Repeat at least 4 times.

FASCIA STRETCHING SEQUENCE FOR THE FEET

As I explained earlier, feet and hands are the two areas that cause the most constant chronic pain. This exercise is designed to relieve foot and ankle pain. For pain relief, we must isolate each individual joint in the feet, helping them move effortlessly and with strength and power. This exercise is designed to work each joint from the toes through into your ankle. Take your time to break up tight connective tissue and locked and atrophied muscles. This is an easy exercise that's safe to do many times each day. Instead of sitting while you watch TV or talk on the phone, try standing and doing these movements.

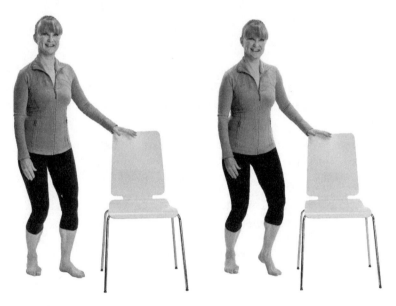

1. Stand facing your chair; hold the back of the chair with one or both hands.

2. Slowly lift one heel. Move one joint at a time—first the toes, then the ankles, and so on. Maintain clean alignment by stacking your toes, ankles, and knees one above the other in a straight line. Don't let your ankle roll in or outward. Clean alignment protects the joints as the weight of the body flows through into feet.

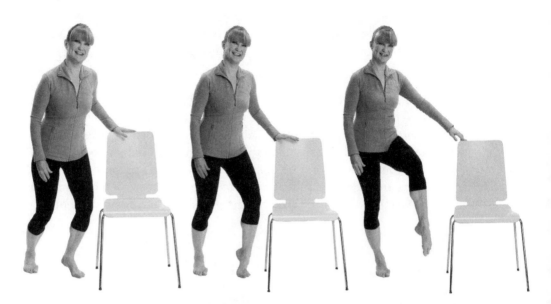

3. Finish by pointing your toes as you lift your foot off the ground. Your toes and the arch of your foot should be pointed as much as possible, which will help stretch your shin.

4. To lower the foot, reverse the movement, going one joint at a time: first the toes, then arch ankles, and finally the heel.

5. Repeat 8 times on each foot.

Incorrect Alignment in Footwork

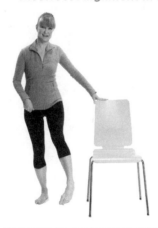

Ensure that you are not twisting or misaligning your ankle. This very common mistake is called sickling your foot, and it causes damage to the ankles joint and ligaments.

LOW KICKS IN ALL DIRECTIONS

The purpose of this exercise is to strengthen the hip, leg, and spine joints while simultaneously lubricating and cleaning them of debris. When you isolate your legs within your hips, you will regain your full range of motion, making many daily activities, such as walking, sitting, getting into and out of bed or the car, effortless and pain-free. The purpose of keeping the kick height low is to avoid using the incorrect muscles of the hips.

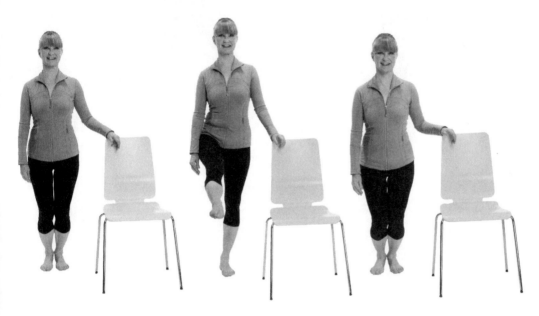

1. Stand with your feet together and your knees slightly bent. Hold the back of your chair with one arm for support.

2. Kick with your knee straight to the front, foot pointed. As you extend your leg, do not let your back or hips move to help the leg lift. Keep your torso straight. Use only your leg muscles—not your back muscles—to lift your leg.

3. Between each kick, return your feet together as you bend your knees.

4. Repeat, making 8 kicks to the front.

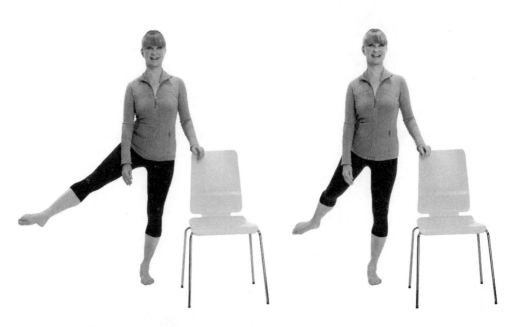

5. Do 8 kicks to the side, returning the feet together between each kick.

6. Do 8 kicks diagonally behind you, returning the feet together between each kick.

7. Switch sides and repeat with the other leg.

· ·

Incorrect Form for Kicks

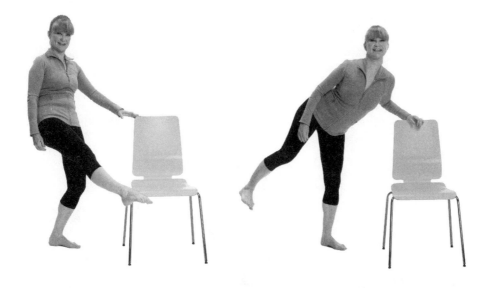

In these incorrect examples, I am using my body to lift my legs instead making the leg muscles do the work they were designed to do. When I am lifting the leg to the front, I am sinking backward, using the lower-back muscles to lift my leg and not my quadriceps. As I bend sideways, the hip muscles—not the abductors—lift the leg sideways. This leads to weakening and atrophy of the abductors and arthritic hip pain.

In correct form, by keeping your torso straight, you are forced to engage your leg muscles. Human beings instinctively try to find the easiest way to move, but often the easiest way ends up in disuse, which weakens muscles. Weak muscles cause pain!

· ·

SEATED SPINE STRETCH

This is a wonderful exercise to rebalance, liberate, and strengthen all of the muscles of the spine. Note: If your hamstrings or back muscles are tight, sit on a riser or a thick folded blanket (something firm) and *bend* your knees. (Do not use a cushion; it will not offer sufficient support.)

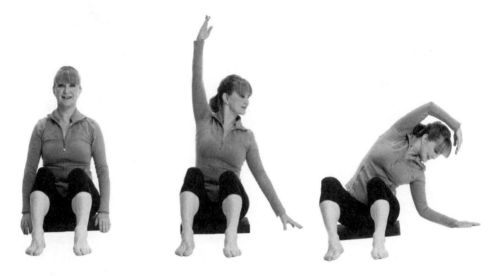

1. Sit with a straight back, your knees bent in front, and your feet slightly apart and flat on the ground.
2. Place one hand on the floor beside you; lift the other arm above your head, elbow near the ear.
3. Bend your entire torso sideways while simultaneously wrapping the upper arm over your head.
4. Bend farther sideways, and sweep the arm in a semicircle from your side around the front and over your feet.
5. Try to straighten your knees as much possible.
6. Finish the stretch by reaching both arms in front, over your feet.
7. Slowly roll up one vertebra at a time, finishing in your starting position.
8. Repeat 4 times, alternating sides each time.

Incorrect Seated Spine Stretch

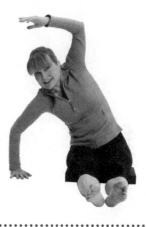

1. Be mindful of your supporting arm. Do not lift the elbow up, as it will block the ability to move your spine.

2. Try to keep your raised arm straight. You may have tight triceps, which makes straightening impossible.

3. Try to keep your arm beside your ear. You might have tight pectoral muscles, which makes lifting the arm beside your ear impossible.

CHAPTER 14

The Stress Workout

As a young woman, Betty Ng raced along a straight path marked by effort, focus, and ambition. Talent and dedication to work translated into scholarships that carried Betty through college and graduate school. She started her career at the top, working between London's financial district and New York City's Wall Street. Her coveted job came with first-class travel and a salary that most of us can only dream of—until illness and pain destroyed her perfect world.

"I was living a very good life," Betty recalled. "The pain was like a surprise guest that disrupted and ruined my party." That uninvited guest clung to her for more than ten years, progressively destroying her life with each additional illness. Her multiple ailments led her to all manner of healers, including top New York City doctors, a shaman in Peru, and meditation masters in British Columbia. She finally found two practices that led her to a full recovery: the ancient Chinese system of qigong and Essentrics.

The pain started in her early thirties when she was one of a five-person team managing a billion-dollar hedge fund. It was the kind of job that required a good night's sleep, but Betty was plagued with severe heartburn that kept her awake all night. The stress of working, combined with lack of sleep, put strain on her body.

Betty progressed through the ranks of prestigious doctors until finally being treated by the number one gastroenterologist in New York City. He ordered many tests at a facility he partially owned; the expensive tests generated results that Betty already knew—that she had acid reflux and a stomach hernia. "When I experienced side effects from medication, he prescribed additional meds to offset the side effects," she said. She saw that she was going down the path of dependence on medications, and she felt she was too young for that.

Medication was the only option her doctor offered. When Betty told him that she had revamped her diet, eliminating alcohol and caffeine while adding whole grains such as quinoa, the doctor asked her what quinoa was. "I was shocked," Betty said. "I would not expect an average doctor to know about these grains, but I thought a top gastroenterologist should. I decided not to go back to him."

And so began a long and expensive journey to seek a cure. Among the health-care practitioners Betty turned to were a chiropractor specializing in applied kinesiology and an acupuncturist. At the point when her digestive issues showed some signs of improvement, she began experiencing back pain, then shoulder and neck pain along with hip pain. Pain would flare up in different areas, ease for a time, and then resurface. She was in a downward spiral, she said, highlighted only by migrating pain.

Her social life vanished as she spent her time either at work or in treatments. "For the first time, I was not in control," Betty said. "When you are in pain and nothing seems to help, it creates a primal fear because you really feel you have lost control of yourself, your body. You have gone from being healthy to being taken over by pain. It's as if your identity, your sense of self has become obliterated."

It was a slow, painful decade for Betty as her health declined into an unmanageable swamp of pain and fear. "I was holding the emotional stress within the body," she said. "It was all tension from the stress and worry of work. Going back and forth from work to doctors all the time just added to the cycle of stress, frustration, and anxiety."

At work, Betty tried to maintain a healthy facade, which only added to her anxiety. She and her coworkers, all high achievers, closely followed the global financial markets that operate almost around the clock, always tethered to their phones. She also traveled a great deal, which was exhausting. Hers was a world in which mistakes could cost millions and were easily spotted by both friends and foes. The need for fast and accurate decisions was constant. "I had a solid track record of making very good decisions and consistently generating profits. I had the respect of my peers, but the relentless pressure to keep doing better and better and never stop, in a very volatile environment, was breaking me," Betty recalled.

All the while Betty's marriage was dissolving. "I actually felt that my pain was causing marital stress because it was so hard for my husband to understand what I was going through," she explained. "Pain can wreck a relationship." She and her ex-husband remain good friends, but at the time the sadness of having to confront the end of her marriage added another layer of emotional stress.

Betty's health had declined to such a degree that she decided to take a two-year rehabilitation sabbatical. A year into her sabbatical, her health had still not improved. By then she'd lost more than fifteen pounds from her already tiny frame. Her digestive problems persisted, and widespread pain left her weak and semi-immobilized.

"My lower spine was so rigid that I could not lie flat on the bed even with a very good mattress," Betty recalled. "The chiropractor took some X-rays and he said, 'You have lost the curvature of your lower back. It is straight.' I asked him how that could have happened. He said, 'I'm not sure.' I asked him the remedy. He said, 'Well, the damage is done—there is no way to cure it.'" Her acupuncturist was more optimistic but felt it would take a long time before her spine got any better.

Betty was desperate. When friends raved about the healing powers of a certain shaman, she traveled to southeastern Peru to be treated by him and his crystals. (Didn't work.) She also explored mindfulness meditation, and went on a ten-day retreat during which she sat in complete stillness for eighteen hours a day. "My concentration to block out the pain got better, but my pain didn't," said Betty, adding that she became even more aware of her body and discovered "micropains."

Finally, friends then connected her to a couple in California; the wife was a neuroscientist and qigong healer, and her husband a biologist and qigong teacher. Qigong (pronounced "chee gung") is an ancient Chinese practice that integrates physical postures, breathing techniques, and focused intention. *Qi* translates as "life force or vital energy," while *gong* means "accomplishment or skill." Qigong practices can be classified as martial, medical, or spiritual. Betty felt immediate benefits from both the qigong training and healing, which helped her untangle emotional issues related to some of her pain and her intolerance of certain foods. "Slowly, slowly, I got better," said Betty. She eventually moved to San Diego to work more closely with the couple, and after a few years of working with them, she was finally getting better. "My body was very weak and my pain was not completely gone," she recalls, "but I was definitely getting better, not worse."

Before her illness, Betty had been athletic, participating in yoga, cycling, and hiking. She wanted her strength back but couldn't summon up the energy to do much more than go for an occasional walk. That's when she saw *Classical Stretch* on PBS for the first time. She was intrigued enough to record the program and try it.

"I felt so good right off the bat," Betty recalled. "I started doing the twenty-two-minute program maybe twice or three times a week; it was all that I could handle at that point. On a week when I wasn't feeling so great, I would do just the stress-release episodes, the ones which just entailed floor work, gentle stretching, no strengthening at all."

Within the span of six months, despite some bumps in the road, Betty grew stronger and became pain-free. Relative to her entire struggle with pain, it was a short time. "You have to remember I had been in pain for ten years and going through different treatments before that! And within a half year, I went from not wanting to do any sports to wanting to become a fitness instructor, to teach *Classical Stretch*," she said.

Betty is now focused on teaching Essentrics and on rebuilding her financial health. "My old colleagues can retire; I cannot. My health ate into my savings. I am starting from zero again. I have to think how I can generate enough income to live for the next thirty to forty years—but that is fine. I feel capable," she said.

Stress has been well documented as a major cause of real physical conditions and diseases. It's no surprise that Betty's body was incapable of permanently withstanding the extreme stress she had put on it throughout her life. Very few people don't have health problems when they endure years of stress. When there is extreme stress, something has to give, mentally or physically—or both.

Pain is a message telling us that something is wrong. We are not trained to listen to our bodies, which was why Betty didn't understand what was happening to her as one system after another became paralyzed with pain. Her body was telling her to stop and get rid of the stress, but because she didn't understand what it was saying (nor did any of the health professionals she visited!), she just kept pushing herself as she searched for a medical solution.

Finally, her body took control of her through pain that forced her to stop. Her pain had become unbearable, and she had no energy to move. Her body gave her no choice; it closed down.

In this high-pressure world, our jobs often require us to live unbalanced lives. Such jobs are often fun, challenging, and exciting, making slowing down to live a more balanced life a difficult choice. However, no human can withstand constant stress. There is a reason why there are so many people addicted to anti-anxiety drugs, antidepressants, digestive medication, and opioids. I know many people who do not slow down when they should, ending up in even worse shape than Betty.

Working hard, achieving dreams, and excelling at our chosen careers are the pursuits that make life so much fun—a continuous adventure and a challenge. However, we all must decide when to pull back and give our hearts, minds, and bodies a rest. You don't have to learn the hard way!

This workout is ideal for those who are overwhelmed by stress. Stress creates tension in our muscles and interferes with the functioning of all the systems of our body, from our cardiovascular and digestive systems to our musculoskeletal systems. Stress forces our body to contract, internally tightening our muscles and slowing down the functioning of basic organs. This is why Betty's pain migrated all over her body from one part to another and one organ to the other.

Use these exercises to relax your muscles when day-to-day existence becomes too stressful. They will help relieve the tension in your muscles and joints, and remind you how good it feels to be pain-free.

NOTE: A stress release workout is not intended to build strength. It is intended to release excessive tension in your muscles. While doing these stress-release exercises, you will be instructed to stay relaxed and floppy, like a rag doll. The healing benefits of total relaxation while moving are powerful. By staying relaxed throughout these exercises, you will see a huge change in your tension and pain while enjoying an increase in energy.

ZOMBIE SWINGS WITH SPINAL ROLLS

This sequence is designed to release tension from the torso—specifically the neck, spine, and shoulders. This is a feel-good exercise. Make sure that you allow yourself to completely relax throughout the sequence.

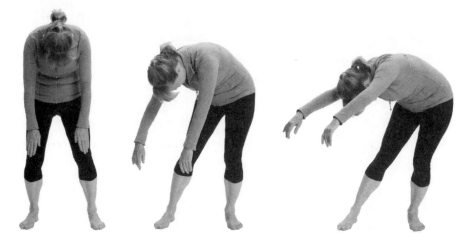

1. Stand with your feet slightly wider than your hips; bend your knees.

2. Tuck your tailbone under and round your back as you bend forward.

3. Dropping your head, arms, and neck forward, allow them to hang totally relaxed in front of you.

4. With your arms and body relaxed and hanging forward, take a deep breath and allow all of the muscles in your arms and neck to relax further.

5. Using a relaxed momentum, slowly sway to one side, keeping your head, neck, and arms relaxed.

6. Let your self sway as far as possible by shifting your weight onto the opposite hip and leg.

7. Return to the center; take a deep breath to *re*-relax.

8. Repeat the same thing on the other side.

9. Slowly straighten your spine, rolling up one vertebra at a time, and finish with your arms above your head.

10. Repeat this full sequence a maximum of 2 to 4 times.

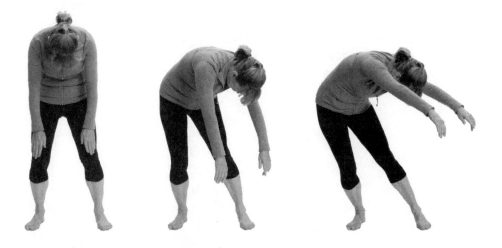

....

Incorrect Posture in Zombie Position

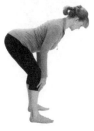

This is incorrect posture. Do not stick out your bum; do not keep your back straight or your head up; this adds a great deal of stress to the spine. Don't support your body by holding your knees, it adds extra stress to the shoulders and neck

Correct Posture in Zombie Position

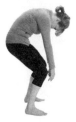

This is correct posture. The full spine is rounded, from the shoulders to the tailbone, which is tucked under. This prevents overloading of the lower spine. Also, be sure to allow your arms to hang heavy in front of you.

....

SLOW SHOULDER ROTATIONS

When we are stressed, we tend to grip all our muscles, and the shoulder muscles in particular. Stress also makes us round our upper back in poor posture.

Good posture requires the shoulder muscles to be strong enough to support a straight spine and flexible enough to be relaxed as they support the spine. So many people hold their tension directly in their shoulders. This slow, deep shoulder rotation exercise is designed to release and relax any shoulder tension.

The shoulders are designed to rotate in four directions: up, down, forward, and back. By slowly working through each of these four directions, you will release any locked tension in your shoulders, neck, and upper back.

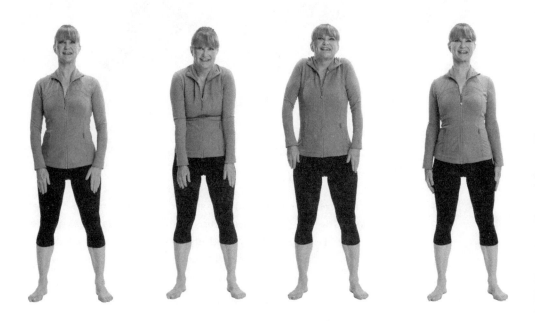

1. Stand with your feet wider than your hips, and let your arms relax at your sides.

2. Keep your arms relaxed and hanging at your sides throughout the shoulder rotations. Do these shoulders rotations smoothly; don't jerk through the movements.

3. Pull both shoulders in front of you as far as possible.

4. Slowly lift your shoulders as high as possible.

5. Slowly drop your shoulders backwards, imagining you are putting your shoulder blades into your back pockets.

6. Take your time to slowly rotate through your entire range of motion. If your shoulders are tense or blocked, take deep breaths to help you release the tension.

7. Allow your muscles to release tension with every move. Give them time to release before continuing in the rotation. Note: If you move rapidly, your shoulders will remain tense and gripping.

8. Repeat 4 to 6 times in each direction (forward and back).

Incorrect Posture in a Shoulder Rotation

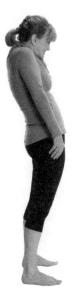

Do not sink into your lower spine; it will force you to round your shoulders.

CEILING REACHES WITH SLOW DEEP BREATHING

This exercise is designed to release tension in the shoulders, neck, and upper back—common areas where we hold tension and stress.

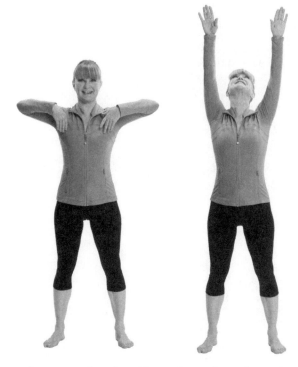

1. Raise your arms above your head and keep them there throughout the exercise.

2. Inhale, contract your shoulders, and count to 6.

3. Exhale and release the contraction.

4. Inhale slowly for a count of 6.

5. Exhale slowly for a count of 6.

6. With your arms still above your head, wiggle your shoulders and upper back, trying to release any extra tension.

7. Repeat until your arms become tired of being held above your head.

RELAXED SIDE-TO-SIDE WINDOW WASHES

Do this exercise in a completely sloppy, floppy, and relaxed mode to break up tension in the spine, bringing pain relief. The combination of relaxation and swaying will bring additional blood flow into your spine, increasing energy and healing.

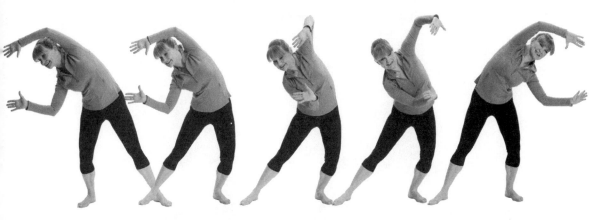

1. Throughout this sequence, imagine that you are moving between two planes of glass as you shift your weight side to side—this will help you keep your back straight and upright.

2. Keep your muscles as relaxed as possible throughout the entire exercise. Imagine you are as relaxed as a floppy rag doll.

3. Keep your elbows bent. Frame your head with your arms and keep your forearms beside your ears.

4. Shift your weight from one leg to the other leg as you lunge from side to side.

5. Let your torso sway sideways as you change sides. Imagine you are swaying in the breeze.

6. Repeat 8 to 16 times.

EMBRACE YOURSELF SEQUENCE

This is a relaxation exercise aimed at releasing tension in the muscles of your ribs, spine, hips, and legs. It also has a slightly emotional component, which adds to the feelings of expansion and relief. When you embrace yourself and rock side to side, it actually feels comforting. And when you open your arms, it feels liberating.

Phase One:

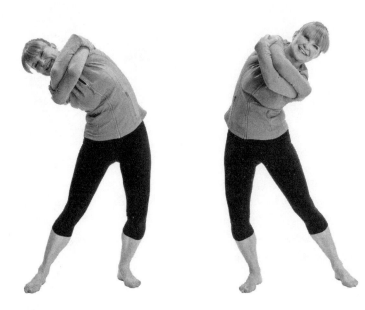

1. Stand with your feet apart and your arms relaxed.

2. Wrap your arms around your body, embracing yourself.

3. Gently rock your body side to side as though you were comforting yourself, shifting your weight from one leg to the other.

4. Rock yourself slowly about 8 times.

Phase Two:

1. Open one arm at a time, reaching for the upper corner of the room.

2. With both arms fully outstretched, look upward toward the ceiling.

3. Pull your arms behind you as you bend your elbows; this will stretch your chest. (I call this movement open-chest swan, because it reminds me of the open wings of a swan. It will give you a feeling that you can fly away, a beautiful feeling of liberation.)

4. Repeat phases one and two at least 3 times.

SEATED NECK TENSION RELEASE STRETCHES

A great deal of our physical tension comes from emotional stress, which causes us to contract our neck, shoulder, and jaw muscles, maintaining the contraction all day long.

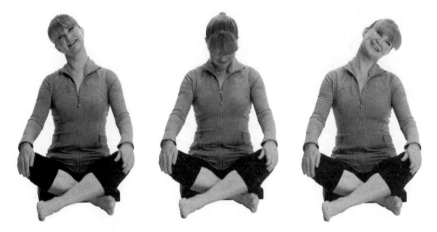

After a period of constant contracting, our muscles seem to forget how to relax. These relaxing movements will take the tension out of the neck and begin a chain reaction of release throughout the body.

1. Sit comfortably on a mat, riser, or chair, with your back straight. Breathe deeply; inhale and exhale 5 times. On your fifth exhale, start the neck stretches.

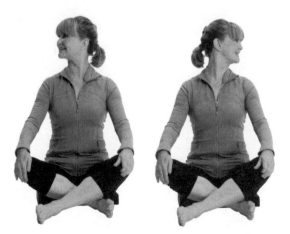

2. Gently lower your head forward; stay there as you consciously release any gripping or tension in your neck.

3. Turn left and right; in each position, consciously release any tension in your neck. Note: When turning your head, make sure your chin is not poking forward or lifting upward.

4. Carefully lift your head toward the ceiling, making sure that your muscles are actually holding your head and that your head is not dropping backward into your cervical (neck) spine.

5. With each individual head movement, inhale before moving and exhale as you arrive.

6. Repeat as often as feels good.

....

Correct Sitting Spine Posture

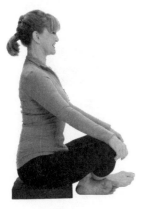

This is correct posture. When you are seated, your spine should always be straight. When straightening your spine, start from the base and roll upward one vertebra at a time.

Incorrect Sitting Spine Posture

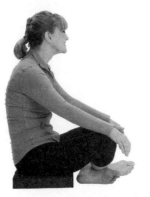

This is incorrect posture. A rounded spine with the neck protruding forward will put tension on neck's vertebrae, creating additional tension. If you cannot straighten your back, sit on a chair or a riser. When sitting on the floor, some people need several risers to straighten their spines.

....

SEATED CEILING REACHES AND SIDE BENDS

This exercise is designed to improve posture. Good posture will improve your lung capacity and your ability to absorb oxygen into your muscles. Again, stay in the relaxed mode and don't work on strengthening your posture muscles. You will be capable of strengthening your muscles much faster after the tension has left them.

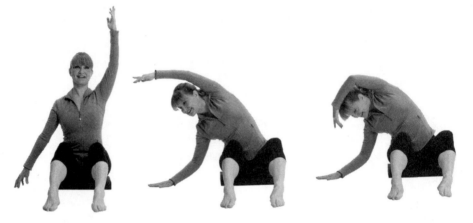

1. Start by sitting on a mat on the floor. Bend your knees and place your feet about hip-width apart.

2. Raise one arm above your head, and rest the other on the ground beside you. (Your hand should be flat on the floor, with your fingers pointing away from you.)

3. Slowly bend sideways in the direction of the hand on the ground; the elbow of this hand should be bending toward the floor.

4. Side-bend as deeply as possible, trying to straighten the arm above your head, reaching toward the opposite wall. (When you straighten the arm above your head, it can pull on the chains of muscles that span from your fingers through to your hips.)

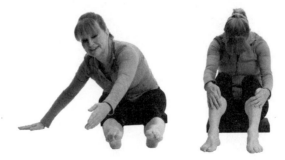

5. When you reach your maximum side bend, wrap your arm over your head.

6. Sweep the arm forward in a large semicircle, finishing with both arms over your bent legs.

7. Gently roll your spine, one vertebra at a time, to return to a sitting position.

8. Repeat on the other side.

9. Continue alternating sides at least 3 times.

Incorrect Seated Posture

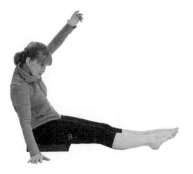

This is incorrect seated posture. If your hamstrings are too tight they will stop you from sitting up straight. In this case, bend your knees to release the tension in your hamstrings; this will help you straighten your spine. Do not compensate for tight hamstrings by rounding your back or allowing your weight to fall backward.

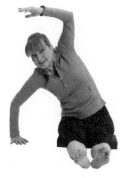

Also, the elbow supporting your body should be turned inward, toward you. When bent, it should point down toward the floor. Pointing your elbow upward will prevent you from stretching your side muscles.

Conclusion:
The Pain Ends Here
and Now

The fitness industry is a multibillion-dollar colossus still its infancy—a blissfully unaware little cherub. As such, there is little existing data on the long-term health impact of many of today's most popular fitness trends. I know there is no deliberate intent in the fitness industry to cause harm, but that doesn't change the fact that many people are harmed by its practices.

The problem lies in a widespread lack of scientific knowledge and the antiquated fitness philosophies behind most programs. Hence the slogans of "No pain, no gain" or "Pain is weakness leaving the body," embraced and chanted proudly by millions of fitness enthusiasts worldwide.

This reverence for pain in the fitness industry has created the illusion that the idea of being fit is synonymous with experiencing pain. Locker-room conversations often involve people proudly comparing their pain and injuries, as if they were battle wounds won in the conquest to become fit. We have been brainwashed into believing that there is only one way to be strong, and that is through the portal of pain. In the sports and fitness industries we have come to accept pain as synonymous with physical fitness and good health.

I hope I have shown you that pain is not the path to good health or physical fitness. I hope you have learned that strength, vitality, and an attractive body are actually found through the portal of a pain-free, flexible, and fully balanced body.

Many breakthroughs have revolutionized modern medicine. Deadly diseases have been wiped off the face of the earth or are now curable. We are living longer than ever before—but not necessarily better. Too many people are spending the final third of their lives in chronic pain controlled by opioid pain medication while being bound to a wheelchair. This is unnecessary; my dream is to change that statistic.

The science behind human aging is relatively new, which is why our parents didn't teach us how to care for our bodies as we grew older. Nor did teachers or doctors. No one knew until recently that a regular rebalancing exercise was the missing link in living a long, healthy, and pain-free life. But we now know, and we can pass on this knowledge to our children and grandchildren to save them from so much unnecessary pain, not to mention trillions of dollars in health-care costs.

It is time for us as a society to develop a more sophisticated relationship with pain. We must recognize what pain is: *a message that something is wrong, a warning to stop doing whatever it is that is triggering the pain.*

Even if you are in pain now, you don't have to be forever. Much of your pain can be relieved and reversed with correct regular exercise. I hope you feel empowered to tackle conditions such as back pain, frozen shoulder, knee pain, arthritis, and fibromyalgia. I hope you are encouraged to know that you no longer have to be saddled with a lifetime of chronic pain—and most of all that you no longer have to live under the fog of pain-relief medication.

Over these twenty years, while developing and teaching Essentrics, I have suffered from many illnesses and needed several surgeries. I have learned the hard way that gentle, correct rebalancing exercise is the fastest way to heal. I have become my most faithful student—because the program works.

It is time for us to be free of chronic pain, to know with certainty that with correct treatment and exercise, most chronic pain can and should be relieved. Pain should no longer be an unwelcome companion that drains us of energy, hope, happiness, and finances. The sooner we deny pain a permanent relationship in our body and take action to rid ourselves of pain through regular, correct exercise and other complementary thera-pies, the sooner we will gain our lives back. Remember:

Pain should not determine who you are.

Pain should not determine what you can do.

Pain should not control where you can go.

Pain should not destroy your relationships.

Pain should not drain your finances.

Pain should not threaten your job.

Pain should not take over your life.

After reading this book, I hope that you now have confidence in your own ability to heal your body of chronic pain. Take charge! Start with one gentle step at a time, and not only will the pain dissipate but you'll also turn back the clock on the aging process, allow-ing you to live well and pain-free for as many years as you have ahead of you.

Acknowledgments

love writing the acknowledgments section because it gives me a chance to thank and highlight all of the people who have helped this book be published. Although my name is on the cover, publishing a book of this complexity would not have been possible without the hard work and dedication of many people.

First, I have to thank my wonderful agent, Ryan Harbage, who is responsible for you being able to read this book right now. Without an agent, it is impossible to find a publisher; without a publisher, you cannot publish an internationally distributed book. Ryan found a home for *Forever Painless* with two of the world's leading publishers: HarperCollins for U.S. rights and Random House for Canada.

It would be impossible for me to fully express my gratitude to HarperWave executive editor Julie Will and Random House vice president Anne Collins. Authors gush about their publishers, and I always thought they were exaggerating their praise. However, after working with Julie and Anne, I, too, am a gusher! These two amazing women published my first book, *Aging Backwards,* and now *Forever Painless*, doing everything possible to support, edit, promote, and advise us throughout the entire writing-to-publishing process. They are an author's dream team.

I chose the subject matter of this book because, over a seventeen-year period, I and my team at Essentrics—Sahra Esmonde-White, my daughter and our company's CEO; Melissa Tran, our chief financial officer; and Lynda Whyte, our director of production—have received tens of thousands of emails about the relief from pain that people experience after doing Essentrics exercises. We have read every single email. We had no choice but to conclude that healing from pain was one of the primary, if not the most meaningful, benefits of Essentrics. We decided that we needed to talk about this subject with our students, teachers, and viewers, even as we waited for the scientific studies to validate what our clients already knew. The material that appears in this book is therefore the work of many years, and I will forever be grateful to these three ladies for the web of encouragement and support and guts that has allowed us to bravely go where few have gone before.

Sometimes timing is essential, which was the case with being able to recruit the talents of Lynn Moore, an award-winning journalist. I was fortunate enough to catch Lynn between assignments, and Lynn was responsible for much of the research during the initial stages of the book. She also used her journalistic skills to conduct the mesmerizing interviews so necessary for the first-person stories in the book. Over the span of her career, Lynn has worked as a journalist and editor for some of Canada's leading newspapers, including the *Vancouver Sun*, the *Toronto Star*, and the *Montreal Gazette*. I will never be able to thank Lynn sufficiently for the contribution she has made to this book.

The gift of having HarperCollins as my publisher is also having Julie Will as my executive editor. Julie brings to the editing table not only her brilliant mind and skill as an editor but also the multitalented Mariska van Aalst. Mariska's magic is expressed as she performs the roles of ghostwriter, editor, and medical researcher. She has an intuitive grasp of what I am trying to say, but she says it so much better than I ever could. Never in my wildest dreams did I imagine that I would be so fortunate to have both Julie and Mariska editing my books.

Writing a book on the subject of healing would be impossible without the consultation and endorsement from people who are highly respected within the medical and scientific community. I have been very fortunate to have several such people as dear friends and mentors: Dr. Helene Langevin and her husband, Ty; Dr. Bradley Bosick and his wife, Lulu; and Dr. Claudio Cuello and his wife, Martha. Over the past years, during many lunches, dinners, and pots of tea, they have encouraged, educated, and guided me into the healing world of scar tissue, connective tissue, and alignment. I owe them all a great deal of thanks for the generosity they have shown me. It is in great part thanks to them that I have been able to develop Essentrics into such an effective, safe, healing workout.

Photography is an essential component of this book. It took a huge team to shoot, organize, and manage the thousands of photos. As usual, Lynda Whyte, our director of production, seamlessly coordinated the entire effort; the results speak for themselves. Annabel Tory tackled the complex task of photo coordination. Her thankless responsibility was to guarantee that the correct model took the correct number of photos. Considering that we needed over five hundred different exercise movements, with multiple angles, it was a daunting job that she accomplished without a hitch. Not one photo was missing!

Wardrobe is also essential for any photo shoot. Our talented marketing manager, Allison Fraser, accomplished this. She made sure we were all dressed in a style that suited the book, in a timeless and simple look. Beatrice Popper did her usual magic on hair and makeup. Thank you, Bea, for your many early rises to happily get the job done.

We were fortunate to have a talented team of photographers willing and able to tackle the grueling schedule: Ian Graham, our in-house photographer; Allison Flam; and Alexandre Paskanoi. I think you will agree that their work is perfection; you will notice that all the movements are well lit and easy to see, which is not as easy to accomplish as most people would imagine. Good job, everyone!

After the photos are taken, the photographers go through a cleansing process, a sometimes thankless yet absolutely necessary technical job done by our in-house graphic designer, Tamara Pettman. Her work guarantees that every photo is crisp and clear and easy for the publisher to reproduce.

Last but by no means least, I have to thank the models: Sahra, my daughter; Pier-Luc Dallaire, an Essentrics instructor and co-owner of a gourmet store; and Pierre-Luc Gagnon, a paramedic by day. I am grateful to them for the hours of rehearsing they put in prior to the shoot; I'm sure you will agree their hard work definitely paid off, as they all look great—and easy on the eyes, if I may say so! No shoot is complete without the energizing of the canteen supplied by Miss Rosie Inc., who kept us happy throughout the days of photography.

When we relate to another person's challenges and see how he or she overcame them, we are generally inspired to overcome our own challenges. I would like to thank Jonathon Powers, Annick Daigle, Anik Bissonnette, Sara Landau, Carol Smith, Sharon Cadiz, Greg

McKenney, Betty Ng, and Paula Hargraves for taking the time and having the courage to share their pain-to-painless stories. I have no doubt that these interviews will motivate and inspire hundreds of people who are searching to find pain relief. I thank all of you from the bottom of my heart.

With much love and gratitude for all your help,

Miranda

Appendix:
Complementary and Alternative Treatments for Pain Relief

ncreasingly, North Americans are looking beyond traditional health care for relief from chronic pain, turning to a host of products and practices that have been grouped together under the umbrella term *complementary and alternative medicine* (CAM). Middle-aged and older Americans are even more likely to make use of natural products such as herbal supplements and mind-body practices such as chiropractic care, massage, and acupuncture. In all, about 40 percent of North American adults use some form of CAM.

Before you engage in any treatment, become informed about the treatment and the practitioner, ask family and friends for personal references, and get information about treatment costs (preferably in writing). Not all jurisdictions license or regulate practitioners of the different therapies. In those that do, seek out licensed ones, or members of the professional body. Always ask for your provider's credentials and clear the treatment with your primary-medical-care providers. In the United States, check out the National Center for Complementary and Alternative Medicine (http://www.nccam.nih.gov). In Canada, where health care is largely regulated by the provinces, check with your local department of health. Limited information is also available on the Health Canada website (http://www.hc-sc.gc.ca). The following are brief summaries of some common CAM treatments that have been promoted for pain management.

Acupuncture

Acupuncture is an ancient therapy and one of the planks of traditional Chinese medicine. It involves the insertion and manipulation of very fine needles in the body at designated points along invisible pathways, called meridians, just below the skin.

The operating theory is that the benefits of acupuncture come from releasing blocked energy, from opening up the flow of a vital life energy called qi (pronounced "chee"). Once the proper flow of energy is restored, the body's natural healing mechanisms can get to work. As we discussed in chapter 2, groundbreaking research suggests that qi may also be related to intracellular communication within the connective tissue, especially the fascia.

Research indicates that acupuncture may relieve pain from osteoarthritis, especially knee pain. It was also found to be effective for neck pain. Some randomized, controlled studies have shown that acupuncture is an effective adjunctive treatment for hypertension, chronic pain, headaches, and back pain.

According to a 1997 consensus statement released by the National Institutes of Health, acupuncture is most helpful when used as part of a multidisciplinary approach to treating osteoarthritis, low-back pain, carpal tunnel syndrome, tennis elbow, and myofascial pain. A 2006 Mayo Clinic study found that acupuncture significantly improved symptoms of fibromyalgia. Overall, acupuncture is one of the most widely used (and well-respected) forms of alternative therapy in the United States and Canada.

Acupuncture is generally considered a low-risk treatment, but adverse side effects can occur. I strongly advise contacting a national accrediting organization to locate a qualified acupuncturist. (See http://www.nccaom.org/ in the United States or https://www.acupuncturecanada.org/ in Canada to find a practitioner near you.)

Massage

Touch-based therapy is another of the ancient forms of medical treatment. Egyptian tomb paintings show people being massaged; in the fifth century BCE, Hippocrates, widely considered the father of Western medicine, wrote, "The physician must be experienced in many things, but assuredly in rubbing . . . for rubbing can bind a joint that is too loose, and loosen a joint that is too rigid."

Over the millennia, many schools of massage have sprung up. The widely available and popular Swedish massage combines long strokes and kneading movements that primarily affect surface muscle tissues. Deep-tissue massage uses more pressure to reach deeper levels of muscles and stimulate lymphatic drainage. Acupressure massage, Chinese massage called tui na, and shiatsu, a form of Japanese body work, also use greater pressure than does Swedish massage, doing so according to the principles of acupuncture. (I have to imagine that these approaches have a similar stimulating effect on the cellular communication of the connective tissue.)

Other touch therapies that incorporate massage include reflexology, a form of foot message based on the premise that the whole body, including internal organs, is reflected in the foot, and rolfing, a structured technique of soft tissue massage that aims to intensely work the body's connective tissue (fascia) and muscles.

Massage is commonly used to relieve muscular tension and to promote relaxation. It can decrease swelling and impaired joint mobility, ease muscle spasms, and increase circulation to promote healing. It can also reduce pain and improve muscle tone.

Massage therapy can be helpful for conditions such as neck and back pain, headaches, temporomandibular joint (TMJ) pain and dysfunction, muscle and joint pain, nerve pain, fibromyalgia, myofascial pain syndrome, sports injuries, and soft tissue injuries. Benefits can include reduced stress, anxiety, and pain along with improved circulation, enhanced sleep patterns, increased oxygen supply, and release of endorphins, the body's natural painkillers. Massage can also reduce heart rate, lower blood pressure, and increase energy and immune system activity.

Be sure to seek out a credentialed massage therapist through the National Certification Board for Therapeutic Massage and Bodywork (http://www.ncbtmb.org/tools/find-a-certified-massage-therapist) or via a recommendation from your primary-care physician.

Chiropractic Medicine

Chiropractic medicine is one of the more common treatments people seek when they have back pain. Although spinal manipulation can be traced back thousands of years, the chiropractic care we know today was developed in the United States in the 1890s by the Canadian native Daniel D. Palmer.

Chiropractic has always been one of the most controversial of the alternative and complementary medicines. In the 1960s, the American Medical Association (AMA) condemned chiropractic as an "unscientific cult," kicking off a legal battle that the AMA lost in 1987. Today, chiropractors are widely respected; they often work in treatment teams with conventional medical doctors, and their services are covered by some medical insurance plans in the United States and Canada. Most people seek chiropractic services especially for back pain, while many elite athletes have chiropractors at the ready. For example, the American Chiropractic Association claims that chiropractors are used by all thirty-two professional football teams in the country.

Currently, most chiropractors do hands-on adjustments called spinal manipulative therapy or spinal manipulation. According to chiropractic theory, misaligned vertebrae can restrict the spine's range of motion and affect nerves that radiate from the spine. These restrictions lead to pain and poor function. Chiropractic adjustments seek to realign vertebrae, restore range of motion, and free nerve pathways. Chiropractors may also use massage or additional treatments such as ultrasound and electrical muscle stimulation.

You can find a certified chiropractor through the American Chiropractic Association website (http://www.acatoday.org/Find-a-Doctor) or via a recommendation from your primary-care physician.

Team of Healers

A well-chosen combination of Western and alternative medicine is often the best way to achieve full pain relief. You might find that the ideal program features help from doctors, chiropractors, acupuncturists, *and* massage therapists. You might seek out the help of physical therapists or osteopaths. You might likely benefit from a warm soak in an Epsom salt bath each night. And you should always include your correct daily fitness regime.

Each member of the team plays a different but essential role in returning the body to full health. None should be excluded as a potential option. We must fully explore and be open-minded to find the best treatment for our particular problem.

Fitness is the one form of soft medicine that requires work on the part of the person in pain. A therapist, machine, or medication cannot substitute for the benefits we gain from exercising. There is no machine, passive therapy, or medication that can strengthen our full 650 muscles while increasing our body's flexibility. The exciting thing about correct fitness is that it can rapidly reverse pain with very little effort.

A pain-free life is entirely possible when we understand how to use the team of health-care professionals—and when we are also prepared to top off their work with correct regular exercise!

Notes

Introduction

1. Centers for Disease Control and Prevention, National Center for Health Statistics, National Vital Statistics System, Mortality File, "Number and Age-Adjusted Rates of Drug-Poisoning Deaths Involving Opioid Analgesics and Heroin: United States, 2000–2014" (Atlanta, GA: CDC, 2015), http://www.cdc.gov/nchs/data/health_policy/AADR_drug_poisoning_involving_OA_Heroin_US_2000–2014.pdf.

Chapter 1: Our Modern Epidemic of Pain

1. Mayo Clinic, "Diseases and Conditions: Depression (major depressive disorder)," http://www.mayoclinic.org/diseases-conditions/depression/expert-answers/pain-and-depression/faq-20057823.

2. M. H. Trivedi, "The link between depression and physical symptoms," *Primary Care Companion to the Journal of Clinical Psychiatry* 6, Suppl 1 (2004): 12–16.

3. S. Mills, N. Torrance, and B. H. Smith, "Identification and Management of Chronic Pain I, Primary Care: a Review," *Current Psychiatry Reports* 18 (2016): 22.

4. International Association for the Study of Pain, "Unrelieved Pain Is a Major Global Healthcare Problem," http://www.efic.org/userfiles/Pain%20Global%20Healthcare%20Problem.pdf; and N. K. Tang and C. Crane, "Suicidality in chronic pain: A review of the prevalence, risk factors, and psychological links," *Psychological Medicine* 35, no. 5 (May 2006): 575–86, http://www.ncbi.nlm.nih.gov/pubmed/16420727.

5. H. Breivik, B. Collett, V. Ventafridda, R. Cohen, and D. Gallacher, "Survey of chronic pain in Europe: Prevalence, impact on daily life, and treatment," *European Journal of Pain* 10, no. 4 (2006): 287–333.

6. H. Breivik, "A major challenge for a generous welfare system: a heavy socio-economic burden of chronic pain conditions in Sweden—and how to meet this challenge," *European Journal of Pain* 16, no. 2 (February 2012): 167–69.

7. D. Lacaille and R. Hogg, "The effect of arthritis on working life expectancy." *Journal of Rheumatology* 10 (2001): 2315–19.

8. M. E. Lynch, "The need for a Canadian pain strategy," *Pain Research Management* 16, no. 2 (March–April 2011): 77–80.

9. R. D. Galloway, "Health promotion: causes, beliefs and measurements," *Clinical Medicine & Research* 1, no. 3 (July 2003): 249–58. Review.

10. H. M. Langevin, N. A. Bouffard, D. L. Churchill, and G. J. Badger, "Connective tissue fibroblast response to acupuncture: dose-dependent effect of bidirectional needle rotation," *Journal of Alternative and Complementary Medicine* 13, no. 3 (April 2007): 355–60.

Chapter 2: Our Living Matrix of Tissue—and How It Can Heal Us

1. E. Krane, "The mystery of chronic pain," TED Talk, March 2011, https://www.ted.com/talks/elliot_krane_the_mystery_of_chronic_pain.

2. H. M. Langevin, "The Science of Stretch," *Scientist*, May 1, 2013, http://www.the-scientist.com/?articles.view/articleNo/35301/title/The-Science-of-Stretch/.

3. E. N. Marieb and K. Hoehn, *Human Anatomy & Physiology* (Pearson, 2007), p. 133;R. Schleip, p. 512.

Chapter 3: When the Matrix Gets Disrupted

1. F. B. Hu, T. Y. Li, G. A. Colditz, W. C. Willett, and J. E. Manson, "Television watching and other sedentary behaviors in relation to risk of obesity and type 2 diabetes mellitus in women," *Journal of the American Medical Association* 289, no. 14 (April 9, 2003): 1785–91.

2. A. Biswas, P. I. Oh, G. E. Faulkner, R. R. Bajaj, M. A. Silver, M. S. Mitchell, and D. A. Alter, "Sedentary time and its association with risk for disease incidence, mortality, and hospitalization in adults: a systematic review and meta-analysis," *Annals of Internal Medicine* 162, no. 2 (January 20, 2015): 123–32.

3. American Chiropractic Association, "Tips to Maintain Good Posture"; North American Spine Society, "10 Tips for a Healthy Back"; and American Academy of Orthopaedic Surgeons, "Spine Conditioning Program," all accessed May 7, 2013.

4. S. Sarlio-Lähteenkorva, A. Rissanen, and J. Kaprio J, "A descriptive study of weight loss maintenance: 6 and 15 year follow-up of initially overweight adults," *International Journal of Obesity Related Metabolic Disorders* 24, no. 1 (January 2000):116–25.

Index

Page numbers of illustrations appear in italics.

About the Author

Miranda Esmonde-White is the author of the *New York Times* bestseller *Aging Backwards*. She is one of America's greatest advocates and educators of healthy aging. She is best known for her PBS fitness show, *Classical Stretch*, which has been on the air since 1999. A former ballerina, she designed the Essentrics technique, which uses low-intensity strengthening and stretching exercises to relieve pain, prevent injury, and slenderize the body. Esmonde-White works with professional and Olympic athletes and celebrities, and teaches classes to thousands of students worldwide each year.